RADICAL CURES FOR COMMON AILMENTS

ROSILAND MILLER

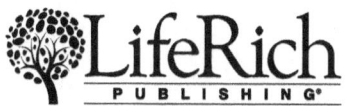

LifeRich Publishing is a registered trademark of The Reader's Digest Association, Inc.

LifeRich Publishing books may be ordered through booksellers or by contacting:

LifeRich Publishing
1663 Liberty Drive
Bloomington, IN 47403
www.liferichpublishing.com
844-686-9607

ISBN: 978-1-4897-3906-3 (sc)
ISBN: 978-1-4897-3905-6 (e)

Library of Congress Control Number: 2021922317

Print information available on the last page.

LifeRich Publishing rev. date: 10/27/2021

CONTENTS

THE REAL DOCTOR'S MERRY-GO-ROUND OF BETTER HEALTH

Having practiced medicine for more than forty years, the Real Doctor comes now as not so much learned as experienced. He brings academia but much more of the practical approach. He mounts the metaphorical merry-go-round of health and lack-of-health and utilizes its perspective to broaden the awareness of physicians and their patients for building strong, healthy bodies and minds. Thus physicians and patients shall better defend against, minimize, and eradicate the noxious elements that slowly and silently or suddenly and loudly rob their health by means of chronic or acute disease. Thus physicians and patients shall build confidence in themselves to grow older and better in the face of an increasingly soiled "nest."

Basically, we're all on a merry-go-round (see Figure 1). Our merry-go-round of healthing or lack-of-healthing (diseasing), however, consists of two rows of "horses" moving in opposite directions. The outer circle of the merry-go-round moves in a clockwise direction. It depicts the elements or forces of Decay, Dysfunction, and Disease that impinge upon or abide within us all. As a composite it represents the sum total of the degenerative, catabolic, and noxious elements that are involved in aging, loss of organ reserves, diseasing, and the untoward effects of therapeutic efforts to combat Decay, Dysfunction, and Disease, and Death. That Cycle of Decay commences before birth in the nature and nurture influences that impinge upon the egg and the sperm and upon the fetus within the maternal uterine-incubator. The Cycle of Decay continues in birth, childhood, young adulthood, middle age, and old age. The mission of the helping professions, of course, is to slow or stop that Cycle of Decay and thus to grow older and better. On our merry-go-round we seek to slow and shrink the "horses" of the outer circle and to magnify and accelerate those of the inner circle.

That inner circle of "horses," moving in a counterclockwise direction, depicts the elements or forces of Repair and Building. It advances the individual toward wellness and optimal health. It represents the operative integrity of body, mind, and spirit that disallows or minifies the encroachment of noxious forces whether outside or inside the person. That Cycle of Repair commences too before birth in the nature and nurture (environmental) influences that impinge upon the egg, sperm, and fetus, as well as upon individuals in young adulthood, middle age, and old age. The mission of physicians and patients remains, of course, to magnify and accelerate that Cycle of Repair in order to grow older and better with a maximum of joy, beauty, and self-satisfaction while also sharing with others the global goals of altruistic advancement of civilization rather than a narrow, logocentric body of thoughts and deeds that merely fuels the motors of the Cycle of Decay for all.

As a physician sits before a patient, the available time spent with that patient is almost never optimal for the task at hand. Yet the physician's prime responsibility is: *primum non nocere* (first of all, do no harm). Too often today, for a variety of reasons, the physician commits more errors of commission than omission. Too often, a too-quickly devised polypharmacy approach is engaged that overlooks so-called complementary-alternative-medicine (better deemed *primary medicine*), a method of care that possesses an arsenal of weapons that slows the Cycle of Decay and that powers the Cycle of Repair through comprehensive understanding of the origins of Decay and the best options out of many considered to fit individual needs.

The four tools of the physician are history, physical examination, laboratory analysis, and follow-up care. None of these, however, counts for anything unless the broad perspective of the diseasing and healthing processes is held in mind. The merry-go-round of life—with all its subsidiary elements—must be carefully considered and evaluated if errors of commission (and those of omission) are to be minimized. For example, the child with attention-deficit disorder must not live with drug therapy throughout his school-life if food allergy is his problem.

Similarly, the adult with chronic sinusitis must not receive repetitive or chronic antibiotics and sinus surgeries if the major problem be leaky gut, yeast overgrowth, and environmental mold hypersensitivity.

The factors that determine the preponderance of the Cycle of Decay or the Cycle of Repair and the acceleration or deceleration of each are here identified as sixteen in number. They are Diet, Gut, Physical Trauma, Infection, Physicians, Toxins, Dentists, Allergy, Exercise, Parents, Genes, Sleep and Rest, Inflammation, Clotting, Glandular, and Mind-Set. I shall comment briefly on each.

Diet: Fresh whole foods, consisting largely of those foods made by God instead of Man, consumed in a loosely rotated fashion, appear to serve best. The epidemic of sugar-related conditions such as diabetes mellitus, low blood sugar, and insulin resistance appears to be tightly associated with abrogation of the principle just given. God did not make refined sugar, refined breads-cereals-pastas, sodas, Gatorade and the like, chips, candies, pies, and cakes. Yet these are the manmade "foods" that commonly displace healthier foods in the diets of too many. Because of the SAD state of the Standard American Diet, largely oriented to convenience, widespread reliance upon a host of nutrient supplements grows increasingly essential.

Gut: The Real Doctor uses the term "gut" to include that part of the body from the lips of the mouth to the anus. The gut thus includes the mouth (oral cavity), the teeth, gums, and tongue, the esophagus, the stomach, the small intestine, and the large intestine extending to the anus. Embryologically the liver and gallbladder as well as the pancreas derive from the gut, hence they will also be included.

The gut, some thirty-three feet in length in the average adult, remains our lifeline throughout life. About eighty percent of our immune system is found in the wall of the gut (the lymphatics) or on its outer surface (the Peyer's Patches). The lining cells of the gut with their delicate secretory capacity to produce hydrochloric acid, bicarbonate, digestive enzymes, secretory IgA (immune factor) and other elements work like an automobile assembly plant to produce final products from a host of components: protein, carbohydrate, fat, water, vitamins, minerals, etc. The gut lining cells are short-lived. They are turned over, replaced, remade every three days. They must "put up with" numerous hazards from the gut contents. Fried foods, sugars, dyes, colors, flavors, monotonous diets and *ersatz* foods challenge gut cells to continue functioning properly when naked-calorie refined and processed foods pour in. Inadequate soluble and insoluble fibers are a hindrance; a "hot- bed" of opportunistic organisms overgrow their space as more friendly bacteria dwindle and disappear. Pesky parasites lodge in cracks and crevices. Various varieties of yeast-fungus crave sweets and carbohydrates and usually find a plethora thereof, but also the resultant yeast-overgrowth from sweet ingestion (and other sources) powers the yen for eating excessive sweets and carbohydrates in general. As the decades mount, the gut manifests its "leaky" nature; its "irritable bowel" nature, its maldigestive and malabsorptive nature. Helicobacter organisms prefer the stomach. Gastritis or ulcers occur. Hiatus hernia ensues. Gallstones and gall-bladder disease join pancreatitis, pancreatic insufficiency, lack of hydrochloric acid, malabsorption of vitamin B12.

Deficient diets having provided a lack of manganese and zinc, proper digestion and absorption suffers. Varied forms of "gas" and constipation abound. Eventually the gut life-line becomes a poor provider. A very strained and repetitively assaulted gut like this over decades often fails to break down food to the desired small molecules. The larger "macromolecules" slip through to cause adverse symptoms within the body and to trigger the production of immunoglobulin antibodies (IgG) that can be detected in the blood as markers of toxic foods or food allergens. In addition, unwanted chemical substances from opportunistic bacteria and parasites often bombard the body.

The gut is our lifeline. A huge and unwieldy organ, it must bear the brunt of all that is swallowed (including the chemicals and particles in the air from the nasal and sinus secretions including the metals from any dental fillings, including any corticosteroid nasal sprays, including any oral medications). Understandably, the biggest portion of drugs sold is for the gastrointestinal tract. Since the central nervous system (brain, etc.) and the gut are very similar in chemical makeup, we indeed have "a gut feeling" about various issues. The merry-go-round concept seeks to preserve, build, and rehabilitate the gut, nearly always by means of natural substances. Major successes are usually seen when emotions, diets, nutritional deficiencies, yeast, unwanted bacteria, parasites, toxins, and allergens are properly envisioned, surveyed, identified, and remedied.

Physical Trauma: Automobile accidents in association with the litigations that accompany them vie with work injuries and their adjudications; moreover an obese, sedentary, and "out-of-shape" population worsens the effects of mechanical injuries. A society that programs its people to expect "compensation" for injury somehow tends to focus on long-term retributive "justice" rather than broader and more effective ways to defend against injury in the first place as well as a differently focused approach to becoming personally well as quickly as possible no matter who pays for that restitution of health. The shared knowledge that patient and complementary-alternative physician bring to bear on both the prevention of injury and the post-traumatic return to health are far more valuable than any financial settlement. Indeed, much of the efforts to restitute one's body-mind "craft" after an assault may well be attitudinal, exercise-related, and involving low-cost dietary alterations, herbal therapies, etc. The Real Doctor does not wish to deny reasonable judgments for traumatic situations. Indeed, the monetary rewards may enable one to purchase merry-go-round counseling that may extricate any individual from the clutches of the Cycle of Decay. Nevertheless, the Real Doctor knows well the force of the circumscribing bands that enthrall the individual whose mind-set expends the vast majority of its energy upon "what I can get" rather than upon "what can I do" to become weller and weller and thus, through time, to deny most or all dysfunction as the result of one's own efforts, not that primarily of a judge or jury. The body is a creature of habit, and the mind must be open if effective problem-solving is to ensue.

Infection: This element possibly may be the biggest "sleeper" of the group. The link of Helicobacter with gastric disease; periodontal disease with atherosclerosis; EBV virus with lymphoma; chronic fatigue, and rheumatoid arthritis; streptococci with rheumatic fever and nephritis; and others awaken us to the possibility that hitherto occult infections may play a prominent role in the diseasing processes for which we have no known origins. No longer can we wait for an acute illness to signal the presence of infection. No longer can we equate the absence of cardinal indicators of inflammation—*color* (warmth), *rubor* (redness), *dolor* (pain), and *tumor* (swelling)—with an absence of infection. A strong index of suspicion for colonization and activity of infectious organisms upon us from the sea of organisms in and around us must be held as a prominent element in the Cycle of Decay.

Physicians: We are angelic life-savers, but we are also devilish troublemakers. The expectation of blind compliance to our authoritarian regimens from patients may indeed give wonderful direction—but at what cost? Nearly all are now aware of white-coat syndrome, a trap in which the office blood pressures are used as the only criterion for placing patients on a lifetime of antihypertensive drug regimens. Retaking office blood pressures with the correct-sized cuff for obese and slender arms as well as utilization of the most placid blood-pressure takers joins accurate home blood-pressure records and honest trials of weight reduction, dietary alteration, and appropriate exercise regimens in order to avoid a lifetime of antihypertensive pharmacology unless truly necessary. A wise axiom for the merry-go-round-appreciating physician is: The best surgery, the best radiation, the best chemotherapy, the best dialysis, and the best medication is that which never has to be used. The Real Doctor revels that we have phenomenal medical interventions. In emergency situations they may have to be used. For less urgent problems, however, complementary-alternative medicine with its merry-go-round perspective promises a much lower rate of errors of commission and omission.

Toxins: Around 1960 Rachel Carson reminded us about our toxic planet. In the understatement of the century, the Real Doctor makes the prescient comment: It hath not grown less. Toxins from industrial chemicals, pesticides, coal-refined generators, nuclear reactors, medical waste incinerators, automobiles, airplanes, etc., abound. Most attention- deficit-hyperactivity-disordered children and many autistics too are toxic. We have available means to identify excessive body burdens of lead, cadmium, mercury, aluminum, antimony, arsenic, nickel, and others. As the decades of life pass, nearly all of us grow in our cumulative burden of toxins from two sources: 1) the external environment including foods and all aspects of modern living such as immunizations; fire-retardant clothing and sheets; shampoos; carpets; antiperspirants; cookware; pesticided homes, lawns and offices, etc., and 2) the internal environment (the gastrointestinal tract) with its load of incompletely digested and absorbed foods, overgrowth of unwanted opportunistic bacteria, yeast overgrowth, parasites, faulty bile secretion, absence of friendly bacteria, and ingested or swallowed toxic metals from the mouth. An inexpensive urine test to detect indican may alert physician and patient to the presence of toxic bowel. Other bowel, blood, and urine tests for various bowel- marker chemicals supply much more information.

Dentists: Like physicians, dentists in general are very intelligent helpers for persons who require their aid. They, however, in general, lack a merry-go-round perspective. Hence they may become hyperfocal in regard to their remarkable skills and tools to construct and reconstruct functional chewing teeth that serve for a lifetime. Like the physician with a prescription-pad reflex, the dentist usually lacks the broad view that the merry-go-round approach supplies. Thus we have dental societies promulgating treatments and avidly defending them when a huge body of information is mounting in a scientific manner that points to the need for change. Fortunately, like physicians, many dentists are now adopting a broader view.

Allergy: The view of allergy as considerably more than IgE-related (immediate allergic) conditions is rapidly taking hold although most traditionally trained physicians in allergy still hold that skin tests for IgE (immediate) reactions are the *sine qua non* for diagnosis and treatment. That may be largely true for the detection of allergy to inhalant substances (dust, dust mites, pollens, molds, animal danders, etc.). A much broader view, however, is required in relation to the very prevalent issue of allergy, sensitivity, hypersensitivity, intolerance, and toxic reactions to foods and the chemicals, sugars, spices, and other accessory food factors ingested with foods. Fortunately, in the Real Doctor's experience, most of the population readily welcomes the wider perspective provided by the merry-go-round model. It finds that delayed food allergies (associated with IgG and other mechanisms) are very common. Furthermore, once identified by elimination diets and/or blood tests, many annoying symptoms and conditions improve or disappear. Those include recurrent infections, stuffed and drippy noses, erratic behavior, fatigue, joint aches, rashes, bowel disorders, bedwetting, migraine headaches, etc.

Exercise: The remarkable popularity of gyms and exercise clubs shows that many are gaining the message of the merry-go-round viewpoint that exercise, appropriate for age and condition, ranks with good food, excretion of waste, need for good air, adequate sleep, and need for companionship as major pillars of well-being. The preponderance of fit individuals in the relatively younger years, however, suggests that many who need fitness to combat osteoporosis, muscle wasting, and the accumulative debilities of advancing years have not yet received the message, or trapped in habits of sedentary living too long, they lack the motivation and support needed to effectively change. A basic concept emphasized by the Real Doctor has been helpful in this regard: Five minutes counts! The message? Get the shorts and shoes on, see to it that the activity—whatever it is: gardening, trampolining, walking, calisthenics, etc.—is engaged most days of the week. Building a more effective program thereafter is distinctly more likely than it would be were not five minutes commenced.

Parents: The Real Doctor here points out that parents are guilty of a sexually transmitted condition: childhood. As such, of course, they are prime agents of nurture, direction, and guidance for our most precious natural resource. Among the other great gifts that parents bequeath to or build within their children, the lifestyles of the parents themselves speak volumes. Unfortunately, with significant exceptions, parental diets today more often turn the Cycle of Decay rather than the Cycle of Repair. The child who is well-cared-for, loved, fed non-toxic food, and taught values by example as well as by precept has a magnificent hope chest with which to enter an increasingly challenging world of information explosion, terror, beauty, and challenge. Unfortunately, today, too often, children may modify the behaviour of their parents before the latter modify the behaviour of the child. Thereafter, it is ever so much easier to go along with pretzels, bagels, cookies, breads, candies, sodas, etc., rather than to face the machinations of a sugared-chemicalized child at the end of a long day or even at its inception. Moreover, those surrogate parents, day-care and/or pre-school personnel, (with certain exceptions), nearly always provide those empty-calorie carbohydrate snacks. Complementary- alternative medicine can invoke great change when parents possess sufficient understanding to slow their own Cycles of Decay and to enhance their own Cycles of Repair. By so doing they can better parent and better educate—shape their own children by more forceful and effective direction but also by interdicting or slowing the runaway trains—the junk-food expresses—of so many out-of-home care-givers and teachers.

Genes: For the present the Real Doctor promotes the merry-go- round message: Turn down the Cycle of Decay and accelerate the Cycle of Repair so that bad genes shall *not* be expressed and good ones shall be unleashed. Do this by the positive manipulation of all the other factors that make up the cycle. For example, the epidemic of osteoporosis and osteopenia (near osteoporosis) attendant upon the graying of America (and the basically sedentary nature of most senior citizens and the difficulty of being well-nourished as the decades ensue) appears to call for estrogen replacement for aging women, yet the estrogen-driving of cancer of the breast constitutes a considerable risk. With a strong family history of cancer and breast cancer too, what to do? Some help comes from the blood ratio of estrogen metabolites, two-hydroxy-estrogens and sixteen-hydroxy-estrogens. We have natural methods to enhance the good twos and decrease the bad sixteens. We shall not wait for the gene therapy to rescue us. Basic non-toxic approaches such as optimal diets and exercise programs as well as effective identification of malabsorption and nutrient-supplement needs loom large and bright in relation to the more reflexive use of possibly carcinogenic hormone "replacements" (although in some cases, indeed, the use of the least toxic, natural hormones or herbs must be employed).

We are fortunate to live at a time when the human genome project is revolutionizing the practice of medicine. Diagnostic tools now exist that can predict which patients are likely to develop chronic diseases, which will respond to a particular drug therapy or react adversely, and finally which nutrients are optimal for each patient's health and well-being. DNA-based testing is available now, and, when combined with functional biochemical testing, an optimally targeted nutritional program for the individual can be crafted. Single-point mutations in the genetic code can now be identified at birth or anytime thereafter in order to favorably modify the modifiable factors for prevention and management of disease. Never before available, such a diagnostic breakthrough promises much in prevention as well as in remediation of current health dysfunctions.

Sleep and Rest: A hallmark of the poorly functioning patient is sleep disturbance. In fact, much of America operates on inadequate or poor-quality sleep. Therapeutic drugs may be needed as a last resort, but many avenues within complementary-alternative medicine are effective. They include inositol, melatonin, calcium, magnesium, tryptophane and five-hydroxy tryptophane, meditation, valerian, and various other herbs and harmless chemicals. At all times, a full survey of the merry-go-round factors of the Cycle of Decay and the Cycle of Repair greatly increases the likelihood of better and best sleep. Those patients who require excessive sleep are especially helped as the merry-go-round physician or patient solves one issue after another to enhance vitality and stamina with improved tolerance for work, thinking, activity, formal exercise, and intimate relations with meaningful others. Again, sleep is so much more regular and refreshing for children when love and reasonable order and discipline fill their days—along with play.

Inflammation: Overt cellulitis and red, warm, swollen and tender skin and perhaps red streaks ascending along lymph channels is relatively easy to detect and manage. Such an acute inflammation contrasts with chronic, low-grade, often occult inflammation that is highly correlated with arteriosclerosis and probably many other conditions. The subtle inflammation challenges the merry-go-round physician to ascertain whence it cometh and how best to suppress it or to dowse its fires. A bevy of natural tools is available and should be utilized before leaping to non- steroidal-anti-inflammatory drugs, corticosteroids, and other medicaments. The high-sensitivity C-reactive protein blood test provides an excellent tool for both the discovery of overt inflammation and for monitoring the progress or lack of progress in management of the condition. The presence of chronic inflammation in Alzheimer's disease—probably incubated over decades—can be at least partially thwarted by chronic, repetitive use of curcumin, ginger, and other herbs.

Clotting: Awareness of the deposition of fibrin and other materials ("klinkers") that impede the free flow of blood through the vessels, especially small vessels, is upon us. Without being formally known as thrombotic disease, this state of pathological clotting often exists for years and contributes to the poor health that many merely attribute to growing older. It can often be successfully managed by the use of heparin and enzyme therapy in addition to finding the basic elements within the Cycle of Decay that trigger the condition. The merry-go-round awareness and evaluation will go far to eradicate the condition. EDTA-chelation therapy with heparin, given intravenously, when appropriate, has long been useful in clearing blood vessels of this impedance to the circulatory flow. Exercise with its strengthening, stretching, and stamina-building, especially with activities that move the lymph within the body (trampolining, for example) are helpful too. Nutrients such as gingko biloba, fish oil (EPA/DHA), garlic, and vitamin E (mixed tocopherols and tocotrienols), as well as the high consumption of watery foods (fresh vegetables and fruits) stand high in antagonizing the formation and maintenance of the state of fibrin deposition within blood vessels.

Glandular: The orchestrated function of the endocrine glands, a symphony indeed, must be fully considered in order to slow Decay and to accelerate Repair. Thyroid, adrenal, gonads, pituitary, parathyroid, and the endocrine pancreas are the organs in question. The hormones themselves that are the "players" in the hormonal symphony include thyroxine, tri-iodothyronine, reverse tri-iodothyronine, thyroid stimulating hormone, growth hormone, adrenocorticotropic hormone (ACTH), hydrocortisone, aldosterone, dehydroepiandrosterone (DHEA), epinephrine (adrenalin), insulin, glucagons, estriol, estone, estradiol, progesterone, testosterone (total and free), parathormone, and perhaps others. The estrogen metabolites, both two-hydroxy and sixteen-hydroxy types, have already been mentioned. Blood, saliva, and urine are used for testing the various hormones. In the case of the thyroid, blood values may not reflect the true state of the thyroid function, hence other methods are often utilized by merry-go-round physicians. The basal-body (axillary or armpit) temperatures of Broda Barnes and its foundation and the insights of the Wilson Syndrome and its proponents have added greatly to the proper thyroid management of untold numbers who otherwise would still be suffering.

Mind-Set: If one harbors the entrenched thought thatcomplementary-alternative medicine merely consists of the "health food nuts" of a generation ago, one denies the very real opportunities for the non-drug prevention and amelioration of misery. Similarly if an advocate of complementary-alternative medicine harbors the entrenched thought that no drug must enter the body lest one be poisoned, one denies some opportunities for safe, effective management of human misery. In the quest for long life and better life, a mind-set of openness and investigation is desired. No one therapeutic modality possesses all the answers for complex human beings living on an increasingly complex planet. Mind- sets that are open and which seek positive solutions that attend to but do not obsessively dwell upon the Cycle of Decay are also most helpful in building better days for one's self as well as others. Desired is focus on what one wants rather than what one doesn't want. Health must be forged with a vigorous mind-set that will not permit the weeds of illness to germinate in one's garden, but also by invoking the reasonable lifestyle that supports that mind-empowerment. How basic it is for triggering that mind-empowerment when one embraces this truism: Disease, for the most part, is not "locked in stone." Most human health departures are malleable, workable, capable of being favorably altered and often are submerged into insignificance.

The primary physician for the graying of America is one who prevents, whenever possible, the establishment and continuation of the diseasing process. He does this by a global awareness of the map of the multivariate factors that cause diseasing. I term that map, the merry-go-round representation of the Cycle of Decay (diseasing) and the Cycle of Repair (healthing). The constituent factors of that carousel shall change as our knowledge expands. Nevertheless, even now, the complementary- alternative-medicine physician can greatly diminish the errors of commission as well as the errors of omission by becoming thoroughly aware of the vast importance of linking together the information provided by history, examination, laboratory, and follow-up visits—all within the merry-go-round model—so as to invoke the appropriate and least-toxic interventions. By so doing, legions of patients shall successfully grow older and better.

The individual patient must learn that in this day and age, if one does not take charge of his health, one shall lose it to the diseasing process. Moreover, he must know that too often also today disease is managed by polypharmaceutical approaches that trigger a cascade of "falling dominoes" within the drug-oriented system. When one drug after another is utilized, when one surgical procedure after another is pursued, when the entire therapeutic arsenal of complementary-alternative medicine is bypassed, ignored, or merely paid lip service, the patient may then be unable to muster the "wherewithal" to invoke the broad outlook and therapeutic approaches of the merry-go-round perspective.

We are all on a merry-go-round of life. By slowing the outer Cycle of Decay and speeding up the inner Cycle of Repair, thus minifying disease and maxifying health, the need for the considerably more toxic interventions with prescription medications, surgery, radiation, and chemotherapy can be significantly diminished. By employment of the merry-go-round concept early in the course of personal care and physician care, the patient will become a more active agent in his own behalf and the physician shall become a broadened and more resourceful problem-solver because of the vast treasure house of resources at his disposal. By employment of the merry-go-round concept, the truism that most disease is not "locked in stone" will become self-reinforcing for positive results.

The Circus Maximus is in every town. The carousel awaits its probing. Enlightened physicians sharing with enlightened patients (as well as vice versa) slow the Cycle of Decay and engage, facilitate, and actualize the Cycle of Repair. In those transactions two ancient maxims are utilized: Know thyself and *primum non nocere* (first of all, do no harm). The inner circle moves faster and faster. The outer slows, slows, slows. Climb aboard. Leave your baggage behind. A new day dawns so each of us may grow older and better with joy to share.

CHAPTER 1

THE POSSIBILITIES

Imagine a future where medicine focused on healing and the prevention of illnesses rather than the treatment of disease, where the medical field followed the concept that the human body embodies the powers of self-healing endowed by nature. With this, imagine our medical establishments' transformation into "wellness" facilities that followed this idealistic concept. As centers of wellness, their basic functions would be the use of the many facets of natural healing and following the concept of "healing without doctors and medicine," preventive health with the underlining belief those most common illnesses, and even serious ones, such as cancer, can be totally avoided. Also functioning as places of learning how to keep healthy, these wellness centers would offer opportunities of learning the importance of individuals becoming more active participators in their own health maintenance, through learning the many facets of self-healing.

Located within natural environments, these healing centers would integrate nature in the healing processes. For example, patients suffering from physical, mental or emotional afflictions could seek healing through fully experiencing nature, such as taking tranquil strolls through gardens, while being led into the art of meditation (a great healer). Filled with flower-strewn lawns, full flowing fountains, huge splendid trees, and comfortable benches for restful meditation, enjoyment of the healing powers of nature would be focused on.

Fresh air filled with carefully chosen healing floral and herbal scents would stream throughout, replacing the typical sterile medical fumes prevalent in traditional healing establishments. Bright cheerful décor, and colors (again chosen for their healing benefits) for instilling a sense of well-being, along with an abundance of wildflowers, plants, and tranquil paintings would fill the setting. Carefully chosen by healing musicologists, music and sounds, such as the singing of birds or the sound of ocean waves would filter throughout, lulling patients to sleep and thus negating the use of sleeping drugs.

For those with health-recovery issues, a diversity of non-invasive healing approaches would be used. Supplements and herbs would replace pharmaceutical drugs, along with carefully chosen hands-on healing modalities such as massage, reiki, acupuncture, spiritual healing and others. For example, meditation would be the standard treatment plan for those recovering from high blood pressure and heart diseases. The objective of following such a regime of preventive measures is primarily to avoid unnecessary heart surgery (a very invasive treatment, resulting in a lifetime of weakness). Included on the staff would be a flock of carefully chosen nurses experienced in diverse facets of alternative medicine. Having certain qualities as compassion and patience, they would be endowed with good communication and listening skills.

In these establishments, specialists in various facets of alternative healing would offer their expertise along with well-stocked libraries having the latest literature on alternative healing. With offerings of various workshops, patients would be introduced to and learn about treatments which they may be preparing to have in the future. This offers a clearer understanding of the nature of individual healing modalities used in alternative medicine, and enables patients to work closer with their practitioners. For those still remaining reluctant to venture into alternative healing, perhaps due to certain warnings from family, friends and family physicians, this kind of preparation will help alleviate apprehension towards alternative healing.

Specialists, who focused on stimulating and regenerating patients' damaged organs by natural means, would replace an orthodox method, which often means surgery. Actually, surgery would be non-existing since variable alternative-healing options would be available and learning about non-invasive healing would enable individuals

2

to make better choices. This includes healing modalities as energy balancing with chakra healing, color therapy, laying on of hands, spiritual healing, imagery, sound energy, acupuncture, massage, reiki, magnetic healing and other affective healing modalities. Exposure to these relatively obscure healing processes to the general public offers healing opportunities that normally would be unavailable outside of such healing establishments.

An important addition to these "wellness centers" would be the research labs, where medical scientists would test the latest discoveries in alternative medicine. Similar to the Mayo Clinic (known for its orthodox medicine and prestigious leaders in their fields), they would gather the most efficient medical scientists and noted healing practitioners in the field of alternative medicine. Unlike orthodox medicine, where medical discoveries are sequestered from the public and data usually only comprehended by medical professionals, the latest findings in alternative healing would be readily shared and translated in laymen's terms. Since this healing is unfamiliar to so many, this is an important issue.

Emphasis would be on motivating individuals to become more interactive with their healing processes, thus becoming more independent. Information acquired through research, lectures and workshops would help individuals better understand the various alternative healing modalities available to them, which would help generate confidence in entering a world of unfamiliar means of healing.

Patients would be encouraged to question, with the expectations of learning something new. In contrast, most medical professionals regard discussing in-depth clinical issues as often lost on patients whose comprehension of medical technicalities is limited. In addition, of course, there's the old adage that "doctors always know best," so what's to discuss? Also, primarily, doctors believe their job is to heal, so that delving into issues, for example, cause and effect of a certain ailment, is close to being a waste of time; they really prefer not to take the time to go in depth, particularly with a roomful of waiting patients. At these healing centers, quite the reverse. Communication would function as a learning process where the many facets of healing are revealed.

BREAKING INTO NATURAL HEALING

Certain visionaries outside the orthodox medical field, dedicated to the concept of the existence of alternative options of healing, were responsible for initiating alternative medicine. As the true pioneers of this revolutionary movement, with persistence they advocated that health maintenance simply meant the adherence to proper nutrition, physical exercise, and positive emotions. However, this movement gradually expanded in wider directions. As alternative healing emerged with certain successes, various medical doctors joined the ranks, using their credentials to endorse this movement's validity. To complement this action, testimonies were growing by leaps and bounds, given by those who, having undergone certain alternative treatments, were healed from lifelong illnesses and nurtured off of prescription drugs.

The benefits are potentially numerous with combining orthodox medicine with alternative healing, particularly for those reluctant in getting into unknown healing processes with healers lacking traditional medical backgrounds.

Many may be disillusioned with their present health care, and are prepared to resort to venturing into something they know nothing of or even further, may relate to as having "witchcraft" leanings. Sickness places us in vulnerable states, where we urgently search out the comfort of the familiar, of what we know and understand. Traditional medicine is more familiar to most. To add, medical insurance companies are less suspicious when medical treatment derives from standard medical care, and from traditional medical doctors. Unspecified healing methods used in alternative medicines always raise questions.

Traditional medical doctors certainly can play valuable roles in alternative medicine. For example, various therapies used in alternative healing require medical expertise to supervise. Chelation therapy, due to its complexity, requires various detoxing programs and dealing with sensitive immune dysfunctions which are best approached by medical professionals. Also diagnosing certain blood tests and other diagnostic tests often requires professional medical supervision. Those suffering from fractures of any kind also require orthopedic and chiropractor specialists. Indeed, while alternative healing has its role to play, it needs to be reminded that traditional medicine also needs to function within our health system.

However, as ideal as it sounds, having medical physicians join the ranks of alternative healing offers no assurance that the end results will be positive. Traditional physicians have been immersed in years of traditional training that is difficult to rid of, and can prove a hindrance, conflicting with methods used in alternative healing. Those endowed with certain skills will be able to cleverly integrate their past medical experiences with their new knowledge of healing. Obviously, this will require certain dedication, creativity and ingenuity. In the meantime, if this aspect of the medical field ever materializes, we may experience a miraculous birth of what the true meaning of healing is about.

FROM A MEDICAL TO ALTERNATIVE HEALING CAREER

One doctor who made a major change from his orthodox pediatrician practice to enter the field of alternative medicine is Ray Wunderlich. Disillusioned by the harsh drugs pediatricians were giving sick children, he found himself arguing with parents that such medicines were weakening their children's bodies and challenging their immune systems. Dr. Wunderlich also argued that drugs rarely completely cure, leaving some children with a lifetime dependency on them. Unable to convince most parents, who were dead set against any "questionable" healing methods that omitted drugs, out of frustration, Dr. Wunderlich sought to change his practice. His mission was to seek healing methods that avoided drugs, for those with fewer potential side effects. This led him into focusing on alternative healing. Unfortunately, colleagues criticized this respected pediatrician, who gave up a lucrative practice to enter the field of alternative health. Critically they referred to him as someone they used to know as a "real doctor," when he once practiced "real medicine." Dr. Wunderlich found himself shunned by the medical establishment he was previously active in for so many years.

Where most doctors have long left their practices, this doctor embarked on a new career while in his seventies; it is rare that physicians practice medicine past the age of sixty-five. Ironically, doctors usually are not the healthiest of people. Statistics claim that longevity is not a one of their strengths, and stress-related ailments are quite common amongst them, which is ironic since of all people, they are exposed to a wealth of scientific medical information. However, Dr. Wunderlich is thriving and continues to research the most recent natural healing information, as his practice becomes even more comprehensive. Unlike most physicians, an expansive medical library surrounds his office. His hectic schedule includes giving lectures and keeping up with a daunting physical regimen that includes running and lifting weights. No doubt, this doctor follows the healthy lifestyle that he preaches to his patients.

ORTHODOX VERSUS NATURAL HEALING

With traditional medical healing, patients either see doctors only when they are ill, and with expectations of receiving a medical prescription to offer immediate relief or being referred to a specialist who usually resorts to some form of invasive medical treatment. Not so with alternative healing; this healing functions more as a means of preventive measures, that is pumping up the immune system to prevent illnesses, which is a gradual process, but resulting in minimizing the impact when illness does occur. Thus, healers are relied on as much for preventing illnesses as for healing. An alternative healing approach attempts to vitalize patients' overall system, making them healthier, which may simply mean including following a healthy diet, exercise, supplements and partaking of various natural healing treatments, thus helping to facilitate healing as being more permanent through promoting overall health.

Traditional medicine in many ways remains cocooned within methods established centuries ago. In contrast, the constant innovations to advanced improved methodologies in alternative healing have enabled it to surpass traditional medicine in many ways. Viewing established medicine being archaic at times, alternative healers argue that their denial of healing techniques outside of their realm, regardless of their proven records, is unfair and borders on being unethical since the medical establishment's oath is to heal the sick. The question continues that while so much medical science is available, there remain some unresolved illnesses. Hence, those unable to seek relief for their particular illnesses, in desperation, have commenced seeking other means of healing which often lead to some form of alternative healing. Actually, this was the predominant factor this movement initially evolved.

Its purpose—*Healing methods need to be individualized, not categorized, since no human chemistry is like any other.*

Alternative healing's basic concept is that humans are endowed with certain natural self-healing physical properties, which if not obstructed will perform freely. The human body is even capable of functioning under physical duress, but only if the body's immune system is strong. At the same time, if illness has attacked the body, rejuvenation can be prompted with the use of certain natural healing remedies, which do not rob the body's own innate strength.

In essence, healing is integrated within the body's own chemistry makeup, along with the aid of human-friendly healing modalities used by alternative healing methods. This form of healing can be compared to plant propagation devoid of harsh chemicals such as pesticides.

Organic farmers know while such chemicals temporarily kill insects, the plant's natural abilities in warding off pests and diseases are weakened; with careful preventive care, such as ensuring crops are well fertilized and watered, the success of their crops without the use of pesticides is ensured. Even more miraculous is that in time, organic farmers find their crops are strengthened because the soil itself becomes healthier since it has not been depleted from the use of chemicals. It appears the plants themselves share their natural inner strength with the soils they are growing from. It is like some symbiosis system between plants and soil is at work here; just another miracle from nature and one that can be compared to healing the body without the use of harsh drugs.

Alternative healing's basic concept is promoting the body's own ability to heal itself with minimal use of external healing aids, such as medicine and various orthodox invasive healing methods, and the developing of a vibrant immune system to ward off illness. In contrast, orthodox healing rejects the notion that the body is endowed with self-healing miraculous capabilities and argues of its limitations of utilizing any of its own functions during illnesses. It regards the body as passive, and suffering from inertia, thus requiring potent external healing processes in order to recover from illnesses. Healing then becomes totally sequestered from individuals' unique physical chemistry, where their individual chemistries are squashed into test tubes, along with the consumption of copious amount of pharmaceutical drugs. In essence this total reliance on external healing methods weakens the body's own resources and minimizes the role individuals can play in their own healing. When individuals become "in tune" with their own bodies, they are able to play a more dominate and intelligent role in their own healing and thus are far from being passive specimens during illness, as believed by orthodox medicine.

Alternative healing seeks out the diversity of a wide spectrum of healing modalities that are intended to focus on individualized healing needs. Thus rather than using standardized healing processes (one size fits all), healing is geared towards the unique medical conditions of individuals, following the premise that no two human chemistries are exactly alike. In contrast, traditional medicine sticks within a standard format of healing, which is narrow and unyielding.

Since orthodox healing is so familiar and raises few questions, few see reasons for venturing outside its parameters, particularly those not accepted by the safety of FDA's standards. Nevertheless, with rapidly growing medical errors, some life-threatening, attitudes are drastically changing. In the meantime, it is difficult to conceive any medical institution would deny the changing face of medical science. Nevertheless, it does. Rarely do family physicians keep up with the most recent healing advances, instead leaving it to medical scientists. However, when patients are sick they don't run to a medical scientist, but turn to their family doctors for appropriate cures. Unfortunately, this can result in not receiving the most up-to-date healing methods because scientific healing advancements and discoveries have yet to leave the science lab (that is until they are FDA approved, which can take time, longer than any other country), then be available in the doctor's office. Medical research is a continuously changing process. For example, medical science has developed important cures for AIDS, and preventive measures of the spread of various diseases and of course the invention of antibiotics. Medical research demands further probing and beyond the normal scope of medical science, which includes venturing into healing methods never attempted, in search for the most dynamic results.

Still, with the multitude of scientific evidences on alternative healing the medical field remains sequestered from it. It was a few pioneers (not medical doctors), who with certain visions were responsible for initiating this movement. Drawing on respected ancient healing traditions, they integrated them with new healing horizons which ultimately resulted in the growth of the vitality of alternative healing.

While in United States, where medicine is tightly woven with prestigious wealthy pharmaceutical companies, there is minimal incentive for doctors to accept any form of healing that does not rely on drugs. In Europe and Canada, where drug companies play less of a leading role than in the United States, natural healing has more credibility and actually in some areas plays a leading role. Actually such therapies as homeopathy, acupuncture, massage and other healing practices are considered mainstream medicine, while in United States, few are aware of them. However, those suffering from chronic conditions or even life- threatening diseases often out of desperation will seek out alternative healing when their doctors fail. Thus rather than choosing alternative healing as a last resort, for them, alternative healing becomes the first choice of healing.

THE GROWTH OF ALTERNATIVE HEALING

In January 1993, in the *New England Journal of Medicine*, Dr. David Eisenberg and his colleagues at Harvard Medical School published an article on America's growing use of alternative medical treatments. Their research included questioning, at random, 1,539 adults as to their use of sixteen different types of alternative treatments ranging from acupuncture to homeopathy, from mental imagery to massage therapy. Thirty-four percent had experienced at least one of these kinds of treatments, and some scheduled weekly sessions in a particular treatment.

Based on this evidence, it was estimated that Americans made over

500 million visits to alternative practitioners in 2002, compared to 338 million visits to allopathic primary care providers. Of the $13.7 billion spent on these alternative treatments, consumers paid $10.3 billion out of their own pockets. This sum exceeded the total amount that insurance companies paid for all hospitalization in that year. Obviously, these numbers have grown enormously since then and expectations are that even a larger surge into alternative medicine will exist, perhaps as much as several hundred million more patients each year that are taking some form of alternative natural healing. It's agreed that this number will continue to rise as a new generation of alternative healers emerges.

NATIONAL CENTER FOR COMPLEMENTARY MEDICINE

Many alternative healing modalities are becoming recognized by the National Center for Complementary Medicine, a branch of the National Institutes of Health. Some professionals agree that it is fortunate to have on its staff the creative and innovative Margaret A. Chesney, PhD, as its first deputy director, who assumed her duty in 2003. Director Stephen E. Straus, MD, heads the planning, directing and managing of the alternative health research programs.

Throughout Dr. Chesney's career she has designed and conducted original research on the relationship between behavior and chronic illness, what is referred to as "mind-body" relationships. She is particularly interested in stress-related illnesses. This center is perhaps best known for the rigorous scientific research it supports on complementary and alternative medicine (CAM). For example, it offers training and membership grants to conventional medical researchers and practitioners to increase their knowledge and experience while assisting pre-doctoral and postdoctoral students who are pursuing CAM research. It also awards funds to universities, medical schools, and foundations to develop training and curriculum programs for CAM research.

The following are some studies CAM is currently conducting:

1—Identifying cardio-protective antioxidants in exotic fruits
2—Characterizing the active components of cranberry that may help prevent urinary tract infections
3—Investigating the biological and chemical activity in the herb red clover for maintaining women's cardiovascular health
4—Studying the effects of ginseng in relation to diabetes
5—Finding more about meditation through the use of functional magnetic resonance imaging, or FMRI
6—Learning more about acupuncture and pain relief.

Another area of research this center is involved with pertains to the immune system and the concept that "the peak of health" can be maintained regardless of age. This includes nutritionists on staff endorsing nutritional supplements as a primary means of helping support the immune system.

Alternative healing practitioners have their own bible of supplements, some more drastic than others. For example, some believe in flooding the body with supplements to prevent illnesses, while others use a more conservative approach. For example, a basic vitamin regime may include the following: a good multivitamin that provides at least 500 mg of vitamin C, and 50 to 75 mg of all of the B vitamins, 10,000 units of beta carotene and 5,000 to 10,000 units of vitamin A. While this formula serves sufficiently for those who are well, those suffering from illnesses require formulas that are programmed for a particular problem and most important formulated to serve that particular individual.

This attitude differs vastly from pharmaceutical drugs, which are intended more to serve diseases than individuals.

Because of the influence of those persistent to gain control over their own health maintenance, and the growing interest in alternative means of healing, the initiation of the alternative medicine division (CAM) within the National Institutes of Health was able to add to their research some very unknown healing modalities. Although funding earmarked for generating new alternative healing was a mere $2 million to start, just the following year, thirty research grants had been added for research into the following:

1—Qi Gong on reflex sympathetic dystrophy
2—Yoga on obsessive-compulsive disorder and heroin addiction
3—Biofeedback training on diabetes
4—Ayurveda on Parkinson's disease
5—Guided imagery on asthma
6—Hypnosis on chronic pain
7—Massage on bone marrow transplant
8—Macrobiotic diet for cancer
9—Intercessory (when other individuals intervene on your behalf) prayer

Obviously, this list is far removed from the realm of traditional medicine, and CAM certainly was not endorsed by it when first introduced. Indeed, under the cloud of objections from many physicians, it is amazing that such action was able to be achieved. However, expectations are that in the near future, such modalities will become more mainstream, and various doctors will eventually seek them out. The inevitable changes medicine will undergo in the future will ultimately include some of these healing modalities, and traditional medicine may have to resort to accepting them. In addition, while appearing objectionable today, they will become standard modes of treatment. To add, as an increasing number of individuals become cognizant of such healing and begin to inquire as to their availability, it will increase the vibrations, thus opening the doors to such modalities, and in which, revealing such practitioners. Now the question is what miracles have to occur for our medical establishment to become enlightened. Perhaps where the money goes is the way our doctors will go.

(As alternative ways of healing become more available to an increasingly aware public, orthodox medicine needs to be prepared to serve a new breed of patients. The bottom line is that patients will expect their doctors to keep up with the latest healing trends. Within an advancing medical environment, physicians rebelling against alternative healing may appear "old-fashioned" and deemed unfavorable by some. By accepting the validity of natural healing and finding a place to use it within their practice, physicians could offer valuable additional benefits for patients suffering from complex health problems that have proven to be unsuccessfully treated in the past.)

With the endorsement of alternative healing by prominent medical institutions, more government support can be instituted, where grants for research in natural healing could expand, thus enabling additional healing methods to be explored. Most important would be insurance companies' support to cover such healing practices. Although individual senators and congressmen support alternative healing, lacking are enough individuals in power to make the essential difference in our present health system. The fact that some receive kickbacks from powerful pharmaceutical drug companies along with the orthodox medical establishment's control all have their effect on the medical system.

GETTING INFORMATION

As of now, the Center of Alternative Medicine is limited in its direct communication with the general public. Actually few know of its existence. What is required is the initiating of certain programs introducing this office's mission such as in the form of holding workshops or lecture offerings. While there now is a federal office on alternative healing, lacking are regional and local offices providing information on alternative healing resources. Such centers would assist those wishing to connect with competent healing practitioners. Often out of difficulty of finding such resources, individuals resort to more familiar orthodox healing for the mere fact that it is easier and more reassuring. Therefore, alternative healing information needs to be channeled out to those having difficulties acquiring it, particularly in rural areas and inner cities. In these regions where illnesses such as diabetes, cholesterol problems, and heart disease run rampart having easy access to alternative healing information enables them to make their own health choices rather than become chained into orthodox healing because of lack of awareness of alternative healing processes. In addition, such available services would alleviate tendencies towards the existing separatism between individual healing practitioners; in turn generating a sense of cohesiveness, which ultimately would strengthen this movement.

HELPFUL HINTS IN SEEKING ALTERNATIVE HEALING

1—To start, it is advisable to continue with traditional medical care, particularly for those with health insurance. This rule also applies until a competent alternative practitioner can be ascertained, or that health expenses can be handled, since alternative medicine is not usually covered by medical insurance. However, few are aware that certain insurance companies do cover some alternative healing, particularly relating to an accident. It is important to pry out this information because it usually is not obvious. In addition, alternative- healing treatments can be more expensive due to their comprehensiveness. It is a normal procedure for alternative practitioners to spend an hour or two screening new patients, which minimizes the number of patients seen in a day, whereas traditional physicians see as many as twenty-five patients per day. Patients under alternative healing care are not only treated for their physical well-being but their complete makeup is evaluated to determine various contributing factors (mind, body, spirit) that may be causing an illness. This includes acquiring a complete comprehensive evaluation, to determine the most effective treatment suitable for patients' individual needs.

2—Since most alternative healing modalities are relatively unknown to the average public, research is essential. Added difficulty is the fact such information is unavailable through the orthodox medical establishment where most would initially search when seeking medical help. In addition, since alternative healers are not listed on any state medical board, searching for them can be difficult. There are various routes to pursue, outside of the medical field, such as local health stores, health lectures held at bookstores, health stores, health centers; also subscribing to a natural health magazine can offer up-to-date valuable information in the world of natural health.

3—Primary care physicians are useful for blood tests, routine checkups, and anything else covered by medical insurance. Primary care physicians covered under health insurance can diagnose blood test results. In turn, once discovering a potential health problem (and having it paid for), rather than resorting to the routine usually taken by an orthodox physician, an alternative healer then can be sought out.

In the meantime, some very sophisticated means of detecting various illnesses are emerging; these differ from traditional blood testing, which often lets subtle problems go undetected. One new technology is Body Scan 2110. The purpose of this scanner system is to identify non- cognitive biofeedback for 6,000 to 10,000 biological stressors in a patient's life. Once the stressors are identified, homeopathic remedies are used to reduce the influences of these stressors in the body. This system is used for homeopathic detox programs, chronic fatigue factors, lymphatic detoxification, and homeopathic detox for metals, inflammation without injections and pain killing drugs, myofascial issues treated, allergy problems handled without drugs. In the meantime, primary physicians usually do not address most of these ailments, some of which can be quite serious.

4—The Internet as a source for information. Any subject on natural healing can be searched on the Internet and usually includes getting plugged into a national group or an association on a particular healing subject. From there, inquiries of alternative healing centers or practitioners in various healing fields can be found...located regionally. This offers a means of checking out practitioners' qualifications and verifying their certification in their fields.

5—Before an appointment is made with a practitioner, information should be as clear and comprehensive as possible via phone or e-mail. A thoroughly understandable description of healing modalities used by the practitioner is pertinent, and written data needs to be layman friendly. Commercial brochures on healing approaches are not adequate. Ideally information should include background of practitioner, qualifications, associations connected to, exactly what the healing techniques entailed, how used, the number of treatments recommended, and costs of everything involved, as well as various substantial easy-to- prove testimonies of patients who successfully experienced these particular modalities. In other words, proof is recommended, particularly if practitioners are not familiar. To add, fees need to be covered in detail as to what they entail.

6—Go slow at first. Integrating alternative healing with your general health care requires careful decision making such as determining when to rely on orthodox care, or seek out an alternative healer. A rule of thumb, at least for some, perhaps those unfamiliar with alternative healing, is if traditional medicine fails to cure, to seek out alternative healing methods, the most common being massage and acupuncture. However, there are many others to explore. Actually, a growing number of people prefer to initially focus on alternative healing and have even given up their former health care practitioners, while others use both methods simultaneously. For example, some may get a diagnosis for an illness from their family physician, and rather than take prescriptions, or other traditional healing methods, seek out an alternative practitioner for other healing choices such as herbal and vitamin remedies, acupuncture, touch therapy, spiritual healing and various other modalities. Most alternative healers will accept patients' integrating alternative healing with their orthodox doctors, as long as it doesn't interfere with their care. However, rarely will traditional doctors accept their patients seeking alternative healing. Actually, those who do usually are opened to criticism from them.

MAKING CHOICES

(Those willing to put their lives into someone else's hands not only need to be ensured their healer is sufficiently trained, but that they are totally committed and devoted to healing.)

Workout—Listed below are steps to help prepare to enter the world of alternative healing:

1—Determining the level of willingness to make the effort in making major health changes, that entails changing doctors, ridding oneself of preconceived medical concepts, and time required in researching into alternative healing.

2—The level of preparation in partaking of some of the modalities used in alternative healing. List below familiar information on this subject:

3—List any experiences regarding seeking an alternative practitioner. Also, list experiences in seeking such. Where they successful? If not, list why:

4—List any negative experiences with the family doctor, and perhaps how alternative healing may help:

5—Now sort out things; what seems acceptable or is objectionable in alternative healing.

A MORAL ISSUE

Envisioning a future encompassing all healing facets, when once-incurable diseases may successfully be healed, and most important, without the use of drastic medical methods such as surgery and chemotherapy and other intrusive imbalanced healing approaches. Future medicine requires healing practitioners in all fields to look beyond the scope of their present practices. As in any field, diversities of ideas and concepts, different avenues for solving problems exist all around. Any given situation has a myriad of complexities to work with, some old, while others new, where change brings forth innovations.

For example, humans evolve into dimensions that render them capable of surviving within the era in which they live. Today's computer age is an example how this modern advancement is now considered essential for survival in today's technological world. Hence with the challenges modernity brings, medicine can no longer remain within the narrow and exacting formulas of the past. While many dimensions have been added to healing, even wider domains need to be explored. Alternative healing practitioners realize some, at present, but unfortunately, they often appear far removed from what is usually associated with healing. However, such horizons need to be further explored, and most important, translated in terms readily understandable and acceptable to the general public.

Even in our sophisticated scientific age, many illnesses seem incurable. We see phenomenal advances in computer technology that boggle the mind, but in the field of medicine too often, the snail's-pace approach is taken. When innovative healing advancements do emerge and challenge our traditional medical system, they often are faced with criticism. The common saying is "While science can put a man on the moon, why can't it come up with cures for such diseases as Alzheimer, idiopathic urticaria, Parkinson disease, MS, fibromyalgia and even cancer?" This truly is a pertinent question and brings up the fact that in no other time in history is exploration in alternative healing so essential. As our modern age brings on changing environments, shifts in lifestyles and societal changes, and even new diseases, responsibility lies with those in medical establishments and healing fields to be open to new challenges and explore every facet of healing. It is the only moral thing to do.

CHAPTER 2

QUESTIONING THE MEDICAL ESTABLISHMENT

Stirring questions probing the once-infallible medical establishment are growing. For example, such issues as the over-prescription of drugs, overuse of specialists for common ailments, unnecessary surgery, suppression of information regarding commonsense prevention of illnesses and general means of healing such as adherence to a proper diet, exercise, and changing some addictive health habits, and the consistent denial of new and dynamic modes of health care, are variable concerns. Upon summarizing these complaints, a compelling need for initiating changes becomes clear. As the number increases of those losing confidence in traditional healing, the search for alternative healing grows more prevalent.

In the meantime, criticisms line up against various medical procedures instituted by the medical field, one being they are often too imbalanced and unnecessarily drastic in situations where less invasive healing approaches would often prove more appropriate. Stringent focus on medical science over and above patients' individual and emotional needs is an added criticism, where patients are treated more as specimens than as human beings, an outcome of a too technologically oriented medical industry. In contrast, alternative healing's objective is establishing the premise that healing should account for patients' uniqueness, where their emotional and spiritual well-being is integrated into the healing process. When medical professionals treat patients in a textbook fashion, remaining within their medical textbook training, the results can be that those suffering from unusual illnesses are unable to get relief for the simple reason their doctors are not prepared to seek other avenues of healing.

Another criticism is doctors tend not to balance their medical expertise with an understanding of the human condition. Medicine is fraught with critical decisions that often are a matter of life and death, thus demanding cold hard science. But studies show that healing the sick requires more, and it is these needs that need to be addressed. The problem stems from the fact that doctors tend to see themselves more as scientists than as healers, because as medical students their studies were swamped with science courses, where such issues regarding the psychological aspect of healing were rarely addressed.

The results are traditional doctors are often ill prepared to understand issues outside of their scientific medical training. Venturing into the inner workings of the emotions and their correlation with physical illnesses were not part of their medical training.

CHANGING MEDICAL TRAINING

One outlook for medical training advocates the need to introducing a broader, perspective view of science, including the philosophy of medical science, with reference to new models based on quantum physics. Also included would be basic instructions in the history of medicine, with reference to the development of major medical and healing systems such as ancient traditional Chinese acupuncture, herbal medicine and other modes of Oriental healing, as well as homeopathy and healing practices generated centuries ago.

Clearly, certain obstacles prevent the ideals of alternative medicine manifesting into a reality. Those attempting to initiate any vital changes within the present health system face much cynicism; of course, the medical status quo remains set in concrete. Dr. Andrew Weil, a renowned alternative healing physician, claims his original cynicism began when he was a first-year medical student in 1964, and was further reinforced by his experiences on a medical school faculty. He claimed that many of his classmates at Harvard had majored in humanities rather than science as undergraduates because of the disappointing quality of the teaching they were receiving in the basic science courses.

Rather than being instructed in how to think about science and health, and learning general principles of human biology, students were inundated with rigidly difficult masses of details to be memorized, even if not understood, and then regurgitated during the frequent exams. Those with good memories passed, those who didn't, failed. Understanding the medicine and the principles behind it was less of a priority.

Dr. Weil's basic complaint, which he claims will not change in medical training as it exists today, is the omission from the curriculum of such general science subjects as embryology, anatomy, physiology and biochemistry. Students were instead studying various systems of the body, and the first unit was focusing on the heart. For example, a prestigious embryologist delivered a sixty-minute complex, detailed lecture on the embryology of the heart that few students could completely digest. Additional detailed lectures were given on physiology and biochemistry, including one by an anatomist on cardiac anatomy.

At the end of the day, students were fatigued, confused, and certainly not as knowledgeable as they should have been. Too much information in too little time was given; students learned how to retain just enough information to pass their exams, and the rest was immediately forgotten, because little time and motivation was given to mentally digest and retain the information. Rather than being taught, students were filled with difficult medical information that was simply thrown at them with little rhyme or reason.

Dr. Weil added thoughts that ideally medical people should re-evaluate their reasons for entering medical careers, perhaps revisiting the altruistic ideals they initially may had when entering medical school. He also felt that some grievances alternative practitioners have towards orthodox physicians are their tendency towards arrogance and autocratic attitudes and unreasonable focusing on monetary objectives in their medical care.

MORE HUMANISTIC APPROACH

Are there any remedies for change in the medical world? Obviously traditional medicine will continue to dominate until certain predominant considerations are applied. To start, medical education needs to undergo drastic changes. For starters, medical training needs to grasp onto the concept that healing is as much a humanistic act as it is scientific. Too often science gets in the way, thus minimizing the humanity of health care.

Greatly impeding the advancement of a more humanitarian approach to health is the fact that medical students are minimally trained in the humanities. However, it has been argued that the latter offers the potential to develop a more humane approach towards medicine, and balance out the cold realities of the test tube. This fine-tuning of the medical curriculum would integrate the humanities within medical training. With such an approach, medicine can be recognized as being more than a science but as a comprehensive healing field having more humanistic goals.

Some medical schools are adding to their curriculum courses dealing with more humanistic issues such as methods of communication between physicians and patients, seeing patients as individuals with unique health problems, thus avoiding standardized treatment and understanding the connection between emotional and physical well-being.

Robert M. Walker, an internist, teaches ethics to medical students at the University of South Florida. Lois LaCivita Nixon, who teaches art and literature, and David Smith, who teaches communication skills, are all part of this new approach to American medical education. Their goal is to teach doctors-in-training not just about science and technology, but also about human values. In the typical medical school curriculum of fewer than ten years ago, these subjects were not taught. However, some doctors argue that ethics is just common sense, and is integrated into the treatment of patients; others question this position. Dr. Walker adds that studies of ethnic cultures, the arts, music appreciation, poetry and fine literature expand the dimension of one's character and help to develop a better understanding of human psychology. He adds that they also enrich one's scope of life, and potentially develop a worldlier outlook that nurtures a more tolerant attitude towards diversity. The potential of such studies is the procuring of flexible thinking, where doctors grow more receptive to approaching healing concepts outside their boundaries.

Arguments fly back and forth regarding humanities courses being added to an already overloaded medical curriculum. Some comment that such studies are useless luxuries. Others, seeing the light at the end of the tunnel, claim their advantages are evident. Dr. Milton Greenspan, a spokesperson advocating the merits of a broader liberal arts curriculum, says many individuals in professional services dealing with people have little or no background in such studies. He adds that, for him, the study of fine arts helped develop certain sensitivities, made him a more well-rounded and aware person, all of which he believes is beneficial with his relationship with patients. He claims that it balances out his overly rigid scientific clinical occupation, and helps put his medical practice in perspective, admitting his preoccupation with the technical aspect of his career often proved an obstacle when dealing with patients.

Dr. Greenspan believes professionals working in any type of human service should have a background in the humanities, and adds that if physicians insist on treating patients in a clinical manner, a medical research career would prove more suitable, where dealing with patients on a one-to-one basis wouldn't be part of their job. Ideally, a bond needs to generate between patients and doctors, where compassion on part of doctors, and trust on part of the patient exists.

(The following are possible subjects introducing alternative healing into medical studies.)

1—Learning emphasis on mind/body relationships, as well as spiritual healing, and learning means to research in these areas.

2—Learning more completely how mental attitudes affect health.

3—Learning to develop instincts, common sense, spiritual and creative skills, and developing certain humanistic qualities in dealing with those in vulnerable situations such as the sick; being equipped with such comprehensive healing skills would enable healers to determine the most appropriate healing method to use, rather than get caught up with standardized stringent formats.

4—Focusing on areas which instruct patients' practical health-maintenance techniques such as balanced diets, exercise, and the many other natural healing practices, so as to improve patients' overall health.

5—Acknowledging alternative modes of healing and learning means of integrating them into medical practices.

6—Learning best means in evaluating patients' lifestyles and the effects they have on their present health.

LOOKING INTO SOME CHANGES

For alternative healing to become more of a mainstream system in the United States, the attitude towards the true meaning of healing needs to change radically. To start, our present-day medical institutions and educational resources are frozen in a disease-oriented mode. Clinical medical training is stringent to say the least, thus making it near impossible for medical students to glance outside their medical studies. Actually to do so would prove an additional burden to their already heavy load of studies. Lacking the promise of a lucrative field, preparing to enter non-standardized medical careers could possibly lower students' status in the eyes of colleagues, thus resulting in minimizing motivation. Concerns regarding medical status are not taken lightly; recently the University of South Florida's attempts to initiate a chiropractor school were vehemently rejected for the simple reason the university felt its prestigious standards would be questioned.

While alternative medicine offers less secure career opportunities than standard medicine, this field has its own merits. For individuals endowed with altruistic faith in the meaning of healing, venturing into it is meritorious in itself, offering a great sense of satisfaction. On the other hand, those choosing the medical establishment tend to be predisposed toward more practical and technical thinking that closely adheres to stringent guidelines. For alternative healers such restrictions are obstacles in their more creative approach to healing.

Individuals endowed with a healthy imagination, confidence, and competence in their fields are more likely to venture into the challenges of alternative healing. That is why few medical doctors who do incorporate alternative healing in their practice are not struggling young medical graduates (which one would expect, since youth is usually associated with innovation), but more established doctors with years of traditional medical practice behind them.

Reaching a stage of dissatisfaction with their present practice, this breed resorted to alternative medicine in search of redefining the true meaning of healing, while being fully cognitive of the workload entailed, criticisms that they would face, and even possibly being sequestered from the medical establishment, along with other rejections. Arriving at a certain fork in their careers, the altruistic meaning of healing for these healers is more vital than a prestigious medical career, which for them too often focuses more on monetary concerns than healing.

However, settled in comfortable positions cushioned with financial success, which the field of medicine brings, any degree of change can be an a unwelcome challenge, which is one reason alternative medicine often seems to be snail-pacing (surprising since this movement started off so promising a few decades ago). Another factor involved is medical doctors fear approaching any healing that deviates from traditional standards of practice even if they wish to for the simple reason that patients can grow skeptical if doctors offer advice outside the mainstream of medicine, which they can readily understand. Also, straying into the precarious world of alternative health, even only so far as advice-giving, leaves doctors open to possible accusations, even to the point of being sued if the advice offered is deemed harmful.

Thus, the consequence from this rigidness is, while we see new healing technologies emerge, doctors' attitudes and methods towards healing the sick have barely changed. Thus stuck with an unchanging medical institution controlled by a medical hierarchy, orthodox medicine has lagged behind some of today's innovative concepts in healing brought on by the alternative-healing field.

There is no denying that the development of various medical technologies has allowed traditional medicine to evolve in this century toward tremendous breakthroughs in the treatment of serious illness. In this manner, great strides have been made in treating many common infectious diseases, in providing relief from various types of cancer and heart disease, and in controlling hypertension and kidney ailments. We have to admit that many people would have died prematurely, had it not been for some of the miracles of its scientific discoveries and applications. However, the fact remains that orthodox medicine too often falls short in successfully treating diseases and afflictions that are not within the familiarity of traditional medicine. While it is effective in treating results of medical problems it has failed to see the importance of cause and effect of illnesses. Another area of weakness is lack of recognizing the relationship between patients' physical and emotional well-being, and the strong influence the emotions have on health.

Obviously, at this time, conventional medicine, and its drugs and surgery, still needs to play a role in the medical world. Not until there is more acceptance and stronger outreach to the public can alternative healing replace some forms of traditional medicine. Exposure is still lacking in many areas nationwide, particularly rural areas where the average local doctor has minimal interest in anything outside his very traditional realm of healing, and of course, there just aren't the facilities to offer such controversial healing modalities as acupuncture, massage, etc., in smaller communities.

Thus, as it presently stands, alternative medicine is only available to those who can afford it. Those in lower income brackets and lacking means in which to learn about alternative healing remain out of touch. In addition, individuals relying on the FDA's stamp of approval are particularly reluctant to venture into unfamiliar healing fields. Sadly, those for whom it would prove most beneficial, such as children and the elderly, who tend to be more vulnerable to illnesses, are denied access to alternative medicine. However, there are individuals who, taking upon themselves to do their own research, and patiently struggling through trial and error, have come up with beneficial information on alternative healing.

To add, insurance plays a dominant role in restricting the public from availing themselves of alternative healing. The current structure of health care in America is formulated so as not to cover any medical treatments outside the conventional umbrella of the medical field. Seen from an economic standpoint, third-party organizations that reimburse physicians for medical treatment are still locked into the Newtonian medical model as the only mode of acceptable therapy. Those wishing alternative healing need to pay out of their own pockets, and some of these expenses are out of reach. This is another drawback towards the growth of alternative healing.

Another obstacle is research funds for alternative medicine are minimal. Establishments that fund medical studies are reluctant to finance research in alternative medicine without the backup of pharmaceutical drug and insurance companies. The people who set medical priorities and disburse research funds are not interested in alternative medicine; it is not a lucrative enough field. Thus, financial prospects are limited in comparison to research in traditional medicine.

ETHICAL QUESTIONS

Medical fraud scam topped $1 billion.

There is no doubt the medical field is a money-making proposition. When a class of medical college students were asked why they chose medicine as a career, over fifty percent reported that it was a financially lucrative career, another thirty percent claimed being a physician was prestigious, and the remaining few said because they truly wished to heal the sick.

Unfortunately, there is a growing number of reports which include fraud, some extremely blatant practices executed by some prestigious physicians in well-respected medical institutions. Obviously, fraud exists in all types of businesses. However, when it exists in the medical field it is particularly distressing. One case involves the following; twelve Blue Cross and Blue Shield plans, working with the FBI, said they had broken into an elaborate insurance scam. Thousands of patients from forty-seven states were sent to California to undergo unnecessary surgical procedures, such as tummy tucks and breast enhancement, for which doctors filed more than $1 billion of fraudulent insurance claims.

Insurance executives and law enforcement officials said that surgery clinics in Southern California typically paid recruiters $2,000 to $4,000 for each patient receiving a medical procedure. In turn, patients received rewards in the form of cash or discounts on cosmetic surgery and payments ranging from $200 to $2,000 each. Yet even after such a horrendous criminal action perpetrated by what are considered to be our most prestigious citizens, nothing of it is mentioned and the criminals got off free.

A TESTIMONY

Refraining from the use of harsh healing methods, alternative healing follows the concept that anything that shocks the body does more harm than good. Thus, healing approaches less invasive to the body are advocated. Following is a testimony of a woman who underwent several of the most drastic treatments existing in the medical field: surgery. Kitty Nelson has fibromyalgia; she also has suffered nine surgeries, all for different health issues. Tragically, she would not hesitate in having another if she felt it was needed. Kitty failed to see that each surgery brought on a new problem, which unfortunately she sought to remedy with another surgery, and of course there is always a willing surgeon to accommodate her. Kitty admits she is surgery prone, but believes it is the only solution, and brags that she is an excellent candidate for surgery because she heals so well. You can't argue with that because her scars heal neatly and she never gets infections. Her friends expected her to come home healed from her last surgery, but she didn't.

Still walking with a cane and drugging herself to sleep due to pain, Kitty has no idea why she is suffering from yet another problem; however, she is ready for another surgery and she still has fibromyalgia, which in itself cannot be healed with surgery; she still has them. In the meantime, this woman failed to realize that each surgical attack on her body affects the equilibrium of her overall system, and years later, she will suffer from severe consequences that will remain with her for a lifetime.

In the meantime, after much persistence from her friends, she sought out some natural healing remedies at a Wellness Center offering various healing techniques that Kitty was unfamiliar with, surprising since many alternative healing modalities effective in treating fibromyalgia are available. However, caught up with traditional medicine, she had no clue. With someone guiding, actually leading her, which Kitty always seemed desperately needing; no doubt, an attitude developed from being a patient so long in the medical system, which regards patients as passive participators, with minimal say in their healing process. Courageously refusing any more surgeries, and determined to get well, Kitty started on an alternative healing program to take charge over her healing. She started with a series of massage therapies and acupuncture treatments along with Reiki and even some spiritual exercises. Joining a yoga class to stretch her aching muscles, never advised by her family doctor, was an additional approach she took. After several months of diligent work, Kitty was seen less and less with her cane. Even with some prompting from a surgeon, she refused, which was the best thing that happened for her. Instead, she stuck with her less drastic means of self-healing regimen, continuing with it even though the result of her progress was extraordinary. Now her regimen of natural healing exercises is basically intended for preventive measures, to avoid reoccurrence of any problems.

A CLEARER VIEW

(Listed below is a summary of Kitty's experience and can be used as a guide when faced with making a decision regarding surgery. The bottom line is alternative natural healing advocates that surgery should be the last choice made for approaching a problem.)

Kitty was subjected to the traditional medicine concept that includes surgery as a very acceptable means of treatment. This woman allowed herself to get caught up within the controls of the medical establishment, thus becoming a passive yielding patient. Not cognitive of the natural-given powers for her body to self-heal, if allowed to, Kitty resorted to violent and desperate means of approaching her medical problems. To add, it is questionable if this woman needed any of these surgeries, but the bottom line was she permitted herself to be controlled by others.

As a victim of the system, Kitty lacked the knowledge of breaking away, perhaps was unwilling to do so, until others came to her aid and helped her find another means of healing. It also appears Kitty lacked the incentive to think for herself and take control over her own health. There were means for her to learn about alternative medicine, but she rejected them, either because she was reluctant to make changes, didn't trust other methods of healing, or was under the influence of her doctor.

Some rely completely on their doctors (as this woman's testimony indicates) to the point that questioning them would be unthinkable; accustomed to a system that expresses almost an exalted reverence towards the medical establishment, places doctors in near hierarchical positions. However, gradually this attitude is changing. Serious medical errors occur at an alarming rate, with reports claiming that over 60,000 patients yearly are either harmed or killed due to malicious negligence or error. In the meantime, much of this reverence towards the medical establishment has tarnished it.

QUICK FIXES

The consciousness of physicians has often come to conceptualize health care as a system for finding the right drugs for patients to make them feel better, but not always become better. Ultimately, patients' expectations are that they are quickly "fixed" with little effort on their part. The great magician physician is supposed to pull out of his magic bag the right cure that is usually some perfect potion (pharmaceutical drug). Given this quick-fix solution, many patients then continue to adhere to their unhealthy lifestyles with little mentioned regarding patients taking more responsibility in changing daily health habits.

This desire for immediate solution is a reflection of the deficiency of self-responsibility that has crept into many individuals' thinking regarding their health. Obviously, self-care in maintaining a certain healthy regime requires discipline. A good example of seeking quick fixes, rather than healing through self-discipline, is evident with those attempting to stop smoking. Running to the drug store for those well-publicized smoke patches, or other smoke-cessation cures, smokers fail to realize the need for self-discipline in changing their habits.

Those who follow healthy diets, exercise, take supplements and follow other health-related activities are usually not smokers because their healthy bodies do not crave whatever elements cause addictions.

Alternative healing regards any type of addiction or general illness, manifesting from a composite of various disorders, curable. Thus, in situations with patients struggling with addictions, a comprehensive change of lifestyle needs to be followed to deal with the problem; no singular approach will prove effective. This can include (along with the suggestions just mentioned) following such disciplines as yoga or tai chi, along with the consumption of much raw fruits and green vegetables, and substituting high-protein beans or tofu for meat. (Vegetarians rarely are smokers.) Also helpful is joining spiritual support groups, possibly following a ritual of meditation.

Since addictions are attributed to imbalance of the mind, body and spirit all three need to be addressed.

The medical field's powerful claws have attempted to clamp it shut through taking certain desperate actions, such as breaking into various alternative healing practitioners' clinics and the confiscation of their records, along with threats of arrest of those distributing supplements to their patients. Such healing concepts as healing the whole patient, mind, body and spirit, along with the use of various natural healing modalities and herbal medicine, have even been referred to as "witchcraft."

MEDICAL HEXING

(The term "hexing" brings up the subject of voodooism. This exotic cult practice derived from Haiti and has traveled to New Orleans, where it has made its home. Voodoo hexing includes the act of one person putting a hex on another, usually an enemy. The practice is a means of surrounding the hexed person with a negative aura, like inserting needles into a doll to cause harm, a familiar practice in voodooism.)

31

A doctor can, in a sense, put a hex on a patient just by commenting, for example, "I don't know what we can do for your particular situation," or any other negative remark, no matter how subtle. During illness, patients are fragile, and in their most vulnerable state. Such negativities can have devastating effects on patients, where focus is placed on illnesses rather than on wellness, and the expectation of "getting" healed. Doctors tendency to view patients' illnesses through the lens of disease results in this narrow negative attitude. Rather than approaching patients with hope, many physicians use what they term as "being straight with the patient," instead of telling them like it is. Unfortunately, this "honesty" has its consequences; patients can take just so much "straight talk," particularly when their health is at stake. Doctors have emotional powers over their patients and can easily influence their moods, so from the slightest negative attitude, patients can easily conclude the worst.

Sometimes, a medical hex can work in positive manner, perhaps with determined patients who set out to prove the doctors wrong and then proceeds to doing something about it, but such situations are rare, and usually whatever doctors indicate is believed. However, patients' illnesses are focused on more so than wellness. The reason for this is the biomedical model from which conventional medical theory and practice derive makes it very difficult to present a view of the healing system to doctors in training. Its materialism leads to emphasis on form rather than function. The healing system is a functional system, not an assemblage of structures that can be neatly diagramed like the digestive or circulatory systems. No doubt, Eastern medicine has the advantage over its Western counterpart. Their emphasis is on function over structure, thus the result is the ability to accept that the human organism has a defensive mechanism that can be stimulated, long before Western doctors realized that the "functionless" organs of the body—tonsils, adenoids, thymus, and appendix—were components of the immune system.

Physicians are not completely to be blamed for the situation they are in. When medical students finish their preclinical studies and go on to work in the wards of teaching hospitals, they are initially inundated with the experience of illness. That is what they see on a daily basis. Third- and fourth-year students, along with interns, residents and fellows are immersed in hospital medicine, the patients they see are usually the very sick, and often recovery is not even considered. Thus, the patients these young doctors see are truly not the full spectrum of illness and just constitute a skewed sample. Their first approach to the medical field is viewing the very sick. Consequently, this imbalance is carried over into the general approach to healing, and thus perpetuated into the field of medicine.

Ideally, healing of the future, rather than focusing on illness, would emphasize wellness, where health practitioners would act as mentors, instructing patients in methods of keeping healthy. Patients would visit their health mentors for health counseling, rather than just when suffering illnesses. This health prevention method would require today's medical doctors to view their medical practice in a different manner. For example, acquiring more expansive attitudes towards fields not of their expertise, thus referring patients to various experts in the alternative healing field. Ideally, this would mean traditional medical doctors working in conjunction rather than competing with alternative healing. Ultimately, this would offer patients additional opportunities of healing. For example, a patient with high cholesterol doesn't have to be immediately put on a drug and warned of imminent death of a heart attack if this drug is not taken. A cancerous lump found on a patient's breast doesn't have to mean there is little hope of recovery. Instead, attitudes can be turned around where hope is nurtured, and in which healing has many possibilities. Anytime the body is attacked with illness, rather than a cold clinical approach taken, all facets of positive manifestation of hope, spiritual guidance, alternative approaches to healing need to be first sought out. This includes keeping the patient sequestered from negative environments, even family members who are inclined towards erratic worrying. Obviously, expressions of compassion are commendable, but they should be cushioned with a sincere positive attitude that offers both hope and guidance.

As individuals become cognitive of the benefits of alternative healing, and learn to trust it, they can forge into its many facets, discovering for them what's most suitable for their individual health needs. Some may readily embrace the unfamiliar treatments used in alternative healing; however, others, indoctrinated by traditional medicine, may find them difficult to accept. The breaking away to seek out healing methods so alien to one's former beliefs can be challenging. However, those under desperate circumstances often are more willing to yield to whatever promises hope, regardless of how unfamiliar a certain healing method may appear. For example, some patients suffering cancer or other serious illnesses, who finding successful cures from traditional healing, going through the regimen of treatments may be more eager to seek alternative healing remedies because there's nothing to lose. In the meantime, there are many testimonies on miraculous cures of cancer (see chapter nine) where some innovative cancer healing procedures replaced the traditional use of chemotherapy.

In the medical field, research on the concept of prevention of illness is minimal; instead, emphasis is on the care of a disease after it occurs. The Boy Scout adage that "an ounce of prevention is worth a pound of cure," makes good sense and certainly could be applied in the medical field, where doctors instruct patients in preventive measures for maintaining health, and where the focus is on wellness, rather then illness. Medical doctors taking on such duties as health counselors, teaching their patients cause and results of illnesses, and perhaps incorporating in their practice alternative healing methods. Of course, all this could be an up hill battle. Doctors' willingness to integrate other healing sources in their practice may ultimately result in lost revenues and raise skepticism from their patients. However, considering the fact healing the sick is of an ultimate responsibility, exploring all facets of healing is essential, and denial of any would be almost criminal. Ideally, medicine of the future will follow the concept that for every disease there is a cure, and all healing processes adhered to gentle non-invasive procedures that essentially restore health rather than offer temporary relief.

BENEFICIAL COMMUNICATION

Narrowing the gap between medical science and natural healing offers more expansive healing options for patients, thus enabling healing processes to manifest to their full potentials. In situations where orthodox treatments prove unsuccessful, alternative-healing methods need to be considered and become readily available. Most ideal would be that traditional family doctors be informed enough to offer patients with chronic or "idiopathic ailments" (simply translate to the illness is unknown) possibilities of alternative healing remedies. However, trust towards alternative healing methods on part of traditional doctors would be required, and the willingness to admit when certain ailments cannot be effectively approached by traditional healing means.

As individual prominent medical institutions and more medical physicians become acquainted and interested in alternative healing, its growth will expand. The ideal situation would be if the government became actively involved. Although individual senators and congressmen may themselves advocate alternative healing, there just are not enough of those in power to make a difference in our present health system. Given the fact that some find it beneficial to support pharmaceutical drug companies and the medical establishment as it is, heads will not sway towards a new direction. A few straws to grasp onto is the fact gradually more medical doctors are entering into alternative healing, however many of them tend to pursue it with a hectic pace with following their own agendas such as pumping their supplements, promoting their books and health newsletters, or have become TV personalities.

Needed is the dissemination of data on alternative healing that is comprehensive and readily acceptable to the average person. The key benefits of alternative healing need to be as readily available to the public as traditional medicine. Quality natural healing remedies need to fill the shelves of pharmacies, and in some situations, replace some proven- harmful over-the-counter drugs. The most recent findings, the very popular pain relief drug, Advil, Ibuprofen and also some cough syrups, and nose drops, which can be addictive...replace them with quality natural remedies that have little or no side effects. Actually, there should be some re-thinking as to our "friendly" pharmacies not being so friendly, as our typical supermarkets as being not so "friendly." While just about every city block has some kind of pharmacy, few and far between are health food stores or establishments dealing with organic produce or other natural products. Unfortunately, few individuals are even aware of this situation, thus resort to that which is readily available and familiar to them, that is, the corner pharmacy or supermarket.

Thus, one of the most vital issues of the alternative healing movement is communication and the spreading of information. Not until the public becomes more knowledgeable about the alternatives available to them will any decisive changes be made. This requires the cooperation of those involved in healing to be willing to put aside their list of profits and consider the values of healing for more altruistic reasons.

While actively protesting the rein of orthodox medicine may have its advantages, such as refusing traditional medical care, more effective would be encouraging traditional doctors to join forces with alternative healing fields, where each comes to realize the similarity of their causes, "healing the sick." Both need to regard the other as not being a threat, instead accept that exchanging healing experiences benefits all concerned. Patients unable to get relief from their physicians, for example, for some chronic health problems, need to feel confident their doctors not only accept healing methods outside of their field, but are also capable of making referrals to certain alternative specialized treatments. All in all, this requires working together, and above all, trusting and exchanging skills. As Winston Churchill once said, "Being generous is smart, it helps all those involved."

KEY ISSUES TO REMEMBER

1—Alternative healing costs are not covered by health insurance and some can be expensive.

2—Most practitioners are not connected to a clinic, but work out of their own office, therefore they are individually responsible for their overheard costs.

3—Alternative practitioners are not supported, or financially assisted by any medical institution. Research is not under the jurisdiction of a major medical establishment, as is traditional medical research, such as by medical instructions like hospitals and government grants.

4—There are no state or federal grants for training in alternative healing medicine.

5—Alternative practitioners see fewer patients than traditional doctors in a day.

ASK YOURSELF THE FOLLOWING:

1—Are you willing to break away from the FDA and medical restrictions regarding supplement use?

2—What part of alternative healing are you doubtful about?

3—Are you willing to investigate new modalities in healing?

4—How do you think you are presently following a natural mode of staying healthy? Are you willing to add more healthy practices? List below what you may introduce in your lifestyle.

5—Do you clearly understand the basic differences between

Alternative Healing and Traditional Healing?

6—What part of Traditional Healing do you question, and why?

7—Do you understand how supplements, nutrients and exercise are beneficial? Are you willing to follow a regime of a healthy lifestyle?

8—List what you feel is holding you back in directing your life to a full healthy turnover.

SUMMARY

Alternative medicine means the healing of the whole person: mind, body and spirit. An alternative healer evaluates the cause of an ailment and recommends healing modalities, taking into account the mind, body and spirit.

Because of this method of comprehensive healing, healing may take a longer time to manifest.

Research is still going on in alternative healing and while the FDA has not approved of most its healing methods, still much proof as to its validity is available.

Alternative healing requires faith and consistency on the part of the patient. Alternative healing requires altering lifestyles.

CHAPTER 3

NEW HEALING CHOICES

A Comprehensive Approach —An alternative healing evaluation may include questions focusing more on the individual's general lifestyle and emotional well-being than on the health issue at hand. For example, included may be a patient's lifestyle risk factors, and various measurements of their rate of aging, such as tests of maximum oxygen uptake and lung function, which is the best indicator of mortality risk since the lungs are most vulnerable to aging effects. To add, prior to undergoing a specific healing treatment, a patient may be instructed to change certain health habits, such as following a disciplined diet, exercising, and undergoing stress management, along with learning about various alternative healing modalities, and becoming aware of environmental health hazards. Perhaps memory and brain functions are tested, and behavior modification discussed.

In essence, all issues that help prolong life take part in an alternative healing diagnostic evaluation. This may include, for example, advice on relying heavily on antioxidants such as beta-carotene and vitamins A, C and E, a formula believed to boost the immune system. In essence, such a comprehensive health preparation enables the patient to better endure specialized treatment, and helps improve their benefits.

The concept is that treating patients for a particular illness and neglecting their overall physical, mental and emotional conditions can be like putting new wheels on a run-down car. In other words, patients' visits to health practitioners are not intended to focus on specific ailments, but to evaluate their overall well-being. This contrasts to traditional care, where a particular health problem is focused on, while other issues pertaining to the general overall well-being of the patient are overlooked.

In part, conventional medical wisdom is misguided; their healing approach is the curing of all illnesses by physically repairing abnormal cellular systems. Through drugs and surgery, the human system is treated as a clogged-up kitchen sink, where there is minimal notice of the complete makeup of a human being. Some healers realize the key to treating diseases is not through "quick-fix" methods so often used in standard medical care. Instead, treating the complete needs of patients, that encompasses their complete internal systems to determine subtle potential dysfunctions before problems manifest into full-blown health problems is proving more reliable for long-term overall health. Even further, this can include taking into account the invisible energetic patterns that guide the physical expressions of life. Such subtle forces between the physical body and spiritual forces hold the key to understanding the inner relationship between matter and energy, between our bodies and emotions and spiritual thoughts.

ADVANCED FINDINGS

Medical research is expanding in every direction, and new approaches and outlooks towards diseases are being discovered, unknown a few decades ago. For example, one particular study addressed the extreme low iron deficiency among ill people, which physicians automatically assume to be abnormal, and thus prescribe iron supplements. However, researchers taking a more evolutionary approach questioned the reason behind this consistent drop of iron during an infection. It was discovered such a deficiency was not an indication of bodily deterioration as previously believed. Instead, it was a means for the body to attempt to use a natural defensive mechanism such as a means of acting as another potent defense against microbial foes. Bacteria, fungi and parasites need iron to survive, and so the body labors to keep this precious metal from them. This is done by transmitting the iron from the bloodstream into the liver where it is stored until the infection ceases.

This is an excellent line of defense, along with a high fever, in which the body's immune system blocks a microbe's ability to snatch away iron packets from the host enzymes that are ferrying the nutrient to the liver. Thus, when aspirin is given to alleviate a high temperature, it can act as the culprit for snatching iron from one's system. To include the mechanisms of the human body similar to animals, are organized for survival. Obviously, there are deterrents that emerge, such as illnesses and accidents, that require special attention. When we pay this kind of attention to the body's own abilities to heal itself, the healing process becomes stronger and more lasting.

CHANGING MEDICAL SCIENCE

Today's environment is permeated with environmental toxic chemicals nonexistent a few decades ago, thus resulting in producing an explosion of diseases relating to these toxins. To add, the increasing consumption of processed foods is also responsible for altering the body's molecules and chemistry, all harmful to the body. Out of this are a growing number of unique ailments that seem to baffle even the most competent physician. Thus, today's doctors are continuously faced with a diversity of illnesses they have little knowledge of, which ultimately results in many suffering from incurable chronic diseases, sometimes referred to as being "idiopathic," a term many doctors find offensive. What is needed are innovative healing methods more applicable for today's environmental illnesses.

The new breed of healers emerging as part of the twenty-first-century alternative healing movement approach with methods that see the human body as an instructional model from which to acquire an understanding of its makeup and its amazing capacity to heal itself. The theoretical perspective adhered to is based upon the understanding that the molecular arrangement of the physical body is actually a complex network of interwoven fields. The energetic network, which represents the physical/cellular framework, is nourished by "subtle" energetic systems, which coordinate the life force with the body. These unique energy systems are so powerfully affected by our emotions and are related to our spiritual thoughts. Thus more understanding of the deeper connections between body, mind, and spirit, which alternative medicine is based on, is part of the medicine of the future.

Becoming more knowledgeable of the holistic paradigms, such as the relationship between the body, mind and spirit, alternative healers realize when treating patients all three need to be addressed in any treatment plan. In other words, in patients treated for physical illnesses, emotional and spiritual well-being are evaluated as a possible cause. Whereas traditional medicine's approach is narrower, physical ailments are singled out from other concerns. Actually for patients wishing to discuss any emotional issues, perhaps undergoing depression or stress, the standard procedure is they are given referrals to psychologists for help, and informed such issues are not within medical doctors' expertise. Unfortunately, that is so true, because medical education does not include studies that hint of anything outside of physical medical science.

Medical research is a continuous process, dependent upon medical scientists' search for cures of cancer, AIDS, and other diseases, as well as the latest pharmaceutical drugs to cure arthritis and high blood pressure, etc.,thus healing science is ongoing. Obviously many innovative healing methods are yet to be discovered, and clearly can derive as much from the field of alternative healing as traditional medicine. In some ways, alternative healing has taken larger leaps and bounds than traditional medicine, because its avenues tend to be wider and more innovative. Actually, it is patients involved with alternative healing remedies who are often responsible in informing their very unaware family doctors of some particular alternative healing they successfully experienced. But chances are they will be faced with some cynical response, such as comments that alternative healing is unproved by the FDA, thus such healing methods are speculative, even dangerous and based on unfounded research. Of course, this is not true. Much of alternative healing is not only drawn on healing practices founded centuries ago but new innovative research is continuous.

KNOWING WHAT AILS YOU

Individuals who consciously make the effort to understand their physical and emotional health, which is what makes them tick, results in more understanding of cause and effect of any given illness; this self- awareness offers the advantage that knowing causes of illnesses can help better prevent them. Those involved with alternative healing often are more astute regarding their health problems and means of treating them than their own physicians; more in-tune with their bodies, they are more readily cognitive of the most subtle patterns of cause-and-effect patterns of any given ailment. This awareness does not indicate such obvious simplicities as catching the flu because there is a flu bug going around. First of all, means of strengthening the immune system to defend against any infectious disease should be a prime concern. However, cognitive awareness of physical stages of mental well-being involves awareness, for example, of nutritional values in foods consumed, supplement intake, exercise routines, and level of stress implications all of which play a direct role in one's health. However, some of these approaches can prove difficult, since searching for alternative cures is not always readily available. However, avenues are peeking through and individuals searching on their own are able to discover bits and pieces of vital information.

FOCUSING ON WELLNESS

Our medical institutions are focused on disease rather than on health. Just look at our national institutions of health; they are national institutes of disease. For example, there is the National Cancer Institute, the National Institute of Allergy and Diseases, the National Institute of Diabetes and Digestive and Kidney Diseases, the National Institute of Neurological Disorders and Strokes, and so on; instead of such names as: The National Institute on Health and Healing, or the National Institute on Preventive Health Care.

Rather than focusing on illness, doctors could motivate patients in the processes of remaining healthy by changing certain lifestyle habits.

This would necessitate instituting new means of approaching patients. For example, no longer would patients be expected to go to their doctors after they became ill, but would make regular "health" visits as a means of learning steps in health maintenance. Of course, this would mean that doctors would have to take the time to learn some facets of alternative healing to enable them to introduce them to their patients, or at least be willing to refer their patients to those who are in the field. Again, this would require a degree of benevolence on the part of physicians, along with expanding medical concepts, and the willingness to communicate to patients regarding healing methods outside of their expertise. Thus, rather than the established medical field competing with alternative healing, pulling these forces together would essentially benefit patients as a whole.

LOOKING INTO THE EMOTIONS

(Key issues regarding emotions affecting physical health followed by alternative medicine.)

1—The belief system has a very direct effect on physical health. This is evident in the medical field's use of the placebo effect on patients whose symptoms nonetheless improve; the belief the fake drug will help, even when the drugs are only sugar pills, has been responsible for miraculously curing patients.

2—Thoughts can control one's health. Positive attitudes can more readily overcome illnesses than negative ones.

3—Keeping the mind active, and activating the soul, has a direct effect on the immune system.

4—When an alternative practitioner analyzes illnesses, he or she probes into the patient's mental well-being.

5—Keeping mentally active, and emotionally balanced, helps to maintain good health.

1—Attempt to evaluate what mental frame you are in most of the time and how you feel it may affect your health.

2—Do you tend to catch colds or flus when you are under stress or experience major changes in your life? Try to connect these together.

3—Do you feel physically better when you are involved in an active project you enjoy?

4—Are there any unresolved issues in your life which you feel may be causing you to feel fatigued, or just not right?

5—Attempt to evaluate at what times you feel your best, when you have the most energy.

6—List what situations you feel make you feel ill. List below what you feel makes you feel better.

7—When you are feeling ill, do you look back to what stressful situations you were in previously?

8—Do you usually feel depressed when not feeling well or do you attempt to do positive healing things to bring you back to health? What are they? List them below.

9—Do you ever consider exercising or correcting your diet when you feel depressed?

10—Have you considered engaging in spiritual thoughts to lift your mood?

The tremendous influence pharmaceutical companies have through their "generous" financial contributions to politicians has an astounding effect. The struggles to endorse natural healing will obviously have to come from other influences, such as resources willing to defend their beliefs. No doubt, complex work is involved, such as persistence in researching comparative data, prepared to consistently defend benefits of alternative healing, being acquainted with institutions that have already developed such goals, and learning from these models. What is truly needed is the development of a corporation or public institutions that join all those in the natural healing fields. Ideally, sometime in the near future, we may see hospitals, healing institutions, and higher-learning centers completely dedicated to alternative healing, but not until changes occur in the politics of medicine. This communal effort would generate a forum of strength and validity where healers can exchange ideas, and promote at large the concepts of the kind of healing that will predominate in the future.

At one time, illnesses were considered treatable only by medical doctors. Many have come to realize this is no longer true. Alternative healing has spread, and many are learning steps in taking control over their own health, thus lessening the constraints of the medical establishment. Unfortunately, the predominance of established medicine makes it almost impossible for many to have available to them information on the why's and how's of alternative healing. Perhaps, bits and pieces of information spread through the grapevine, for example comments revealing some miraculous treatments experienced through some type of unfamiliar treatments. However, the bottom line is that more information needs to wind its way out to the public before alternative medicine can forcibly stride forward as a predominant means of healing nationwide.

CHAPTER 4

TAKING CONTROL OVER YOUR HEALTH

One objective of alternative healing is motivating individuals to take a more active role in their health care. The usual procedure followed by alternative healing practitioners is, along with any healing process, patients are instructed steps on self health maintenance they can follow. This results in generating a sense of independence on the part of patients. The ability to ward off diseases and other afflictions by being aware of certain self-healing or prevention techniques offers a great sense of freedom.

"Assuming more responsibility for one's own health is becoming quite popular these days. Self-healthcare is something we all should espouse," said Dr. Allen Doumas, associate director of health of the American Association, Department of Education. "It's a great way for people to take care of themselves," he said.

Recent statistics indicate this trend is more widespread than many realize. For example, seventy-five to eighty-five percent of all illnesses in Great Britain are now managed without doctor's consultations. Also, nearly half of all acute conditions in the United States are now being treated without physician care. In many cases it was discovered that, due to the practice of various methods of preventive care, dependence on professional medical care was minimized.

As Dr. Michael DeCosmo from Florida commented in his talk at his clinic, "Taking control over your health includes paying attention to maintaining moderation in everything you do. Allowing something to dominate you, where you have become addicted to something such as eating, sexual activities, gross entertainment, stressful work, etc., results in losing control over your health life. Besides compromising your sense of self-empowerment, this imbalance affects both physical and emotional well-being. However, the key word is moderation, not overt and rigid discipline to follow some health regime, which then becomes a dread or too difficult to follow in time. Seeking good health— physically, mentally and spiritually need not become a horrific struggle, but a journey for achieving a better and longer life."

STEP 1—BECOMING AWARE AND CONTROLLING WHAT AILS YOU

Alternative medicine follows the concept that each medical affliction is attributable to a very decisive cause. Awareness of that cause is regarded as vital; to solve the problem and offer a powerful means of determining what preventive measures can be adhered to can avoid future problems. Thus, rather than just focusing on end results of healing, alternative practitioners scrutinize the basis of an illness. This comprehensive approach acts as a motivator for patients to take steps to become more responsible over their own health. This includes awareness of emotional or lifestyle stressors and their potential negative effects on health. For example, such negative experiences as divorce, a death in the family, losing a job, etc., which cause internal stresses can manifest into health problems. Even entering a new job situation or moving to a new location can be enough stress factors to result in illnesses. Statistics report that college freshman students are particularly vulnerable to catching colds and flus, the stress of sudden change and having to fend for oneself, plus being sequestered from domestic security lowers the immune system, thus, allowing the student succumb to the disease.

Illnesses may be a symbolic reflection of one's own state of internal unrest, or spiritual blockage. While an external situation can be responsible, often an internal imbalance can render the body more susceptible to an illness. Emotional difficulties can readily translate to physiological weaknesses, which can gradually result in a localized system breakdown in the physical body, i.e. disease. When illness occurs, it can indicate that certain subtle energies inside the body, or emotions, either consciously or subconsciously are being constricted.

Patients under the care of alternative healing tend to know more what ails them than their own physicians. In tune with their bodies, they are cognizant of subtleties, and certain changing physical patterns. This along with awareness of cause and effect of illnesses, and continual researching of alternative cures, gathering the latest data on natural healing and healthy lifestyles, keeps them well informed. In contrast, the average medical doctor lacks the time or motivation to seek out new alternative healing methods. However, medical research is a continuous process and depends upon medical science searching for cures for cancer, AIDS, and other diseases, as well as discovery of the latest pharmaceutical drugs to cure arthritis and high blood pressure, etc. Thus remaining aloof towards medical healing concepts outside of traditional medicine can potentially put a halt to some vital research. In many situations, most patients inform their family doctors of the latest healing discoveries. Most often, the doctor criticizes the patient and warns them that alternative remedies are not FDA approved.

STEP 2—MAKING YOUR OWN HEALTH DECISIONS

Your best approach is in acquiring a complete understanding of the health problem; if the suggested approach is appropriate for you, and you have complete faith in the procedure, go with it. I have two doctors that I see. One is my primary care physician, where I receive yearly physicals and blood tests, since they are covered by my insurance,and the other doctor is an alternative practitioner (not covered by insurance), who offers advice on what natural healing remedies I can substitute for any prescription drug my primary care physician may give me.

Their approaches vastly differ from each other. For example, for years my orthodox doctor insisted a diabetes medication was essential and even threatened to drop me as a patient if I refused this "life-saving drug," as she put it. On the next visit to her office, she was surprised I was still alive. I attempted to explain to her that my diabetes was under control; I was following certain measures prescribed in this book. A few months later, I discovered my doctor has taken a leave of absence to attend an alternative healing workshop. I guess she caught on.

STEP 3—LOOK FOR ANOTHER WAY OF HEALING

Physicians emphasize the taking of medical drugs and often use overly intrusive healing procedures that sometimes are unnecessary. A friend of mine, Eric, was balancing several medications for his heart disease each morning, noon and again at night. His doctor kept switching his medication from one drug to another, seemingly using him as a guinea pig, experimenting with what drugs worked best. In no time, Eric's doctor advised him to curb his active drinking habit. The doctor believed the excessive drinking to be the core of his health problems, not the great assortment of medications.

To make matters worse, the side effects of these drugs were getting the best of my friend. His one-time hearty and intelligent conversations gradually became weak and unfocussed; getting the words out was an effort. Attempting to give advice to my friend in his minimizing these drugs caused him to become defensive, insisting that his doctors knew best. However, one day while taking his usual cupful of pills, and almost passing out, he started to listen and even considered looking into some aspects of alternative healing. Eric started substituting alternative cures for some of his drugs and eventually came back to his normal self.

Listed below are precautions for some prescription drugs.

1—Attempt to avoid taking prescription drugs unless in emergency situations.

2—When a doctor prescribes a drug, research its side effects.

Usually pharmacists take a conservative approach regarding side effects of drugs. A book on the subject, such as the *Consumer's Guide on Prescription Drugs* with Peggy Boucher Mullen's "Pharmaceutical Doctor" is helpful. This guide covers important information on hundreds of brand-name medications and their generic equivalents, how to talk to your doctor and pharmacist about them, how to administer the drugs, and coping with their side effects.

Consider the following:

1—If you are taking any drugs, are you satisfied with them? Do you know the side effects of the drug?

2—Ask your doctor if you can substitute the prescribed drug he is giving you with a health supplement. Since doctors know little or nothing about health supplements, you may not be very successful in using this approach.

3—When your doctor prescribes a drug, ask a reputable health practitioner if you can substitute a natural remedy. However, if you are taking a drug for a life- threatening disease, it is advisable to continue using it, but along with it, use a health supplement that will boost your immune system to minimize the recovery length of the illness.

4—I recommend that in flu season, you stock your medicine cabinet with the following supplements for fast recovery and in help preventing the disease: vitamin C, echinacea, and elderberry. There is a good product for boosting the immune system, and also fending off colds and flus, called Sambucol, which is available in most health stores. However, your doctor will probably know nothing about it.

5—Attempt to substitute alternative supplements, homeopathic remedies or Chinese herbs for all over-the-counter drugs, and watch out for household cleaning and beauty products like deodorant, face creams, and makeup, since they all contain synthetic chemicals, some with harmful effects to the health. Many brands of mouthwashes have alcohol, even in children's products, and many deodorants contain cancer- producing aluminum, which has also been linked to Alzheimer's disease.

STEP 4—RESEARCH, LEARN, BECOME YOUR OWN HEALER

Search out every possible treatment available. Much information is now available. Bookstores are stocked with the latest on alternative healing and these selections are expanding; new information is always emerging. However, watch out for those promising quick fixes, making claims they can cure everything, particularly with unfamiliar remedies. Just like in any field, the alternative healing field has its charlatans, which is particularly unfortunate since some, after being disappointed with conventional medicine, look to it as a "saving grace." In addition, there are the "naysayers" who are ready to criticize any alternative formula or supplement.

STEP 5—MAKE CONSTRUCTIVE FRIENDSHIPS WITH HEALTH PRACTITIONERS

Since writing this book, scores of healers, in all walks of natural healing, eagerly shared their expertise and offered to explain some very complex therapies. Compiling the material in this book has taken many years of searching, and discussing the therapies with these willing professionals. I believe mutual respect and interest nurtured some camaraderie in giving enormous valuable firsthand information, for which I am most grateful.

STEP 6—MAKING RADICAL CHANGES

Since past generations knew little of alternative healing, it left many having to forge ahead on their own searching for information. For centuries, people had no other resource but to turn to the medical establishment. Thus, today, the tragedy is children suffering from illnesses such as diabetes and cholesterol from poor eating habits come from families whose knowledge often is minimal in such simple issues as healthy eating along with commonsense healthy living and nothing at all about natural healing. Thus, they need to be dependant on their medical doctors to cure them. Thus as it now stands, alternative medicine is far from being a household name.

This new outlook on healing is difficult to understand and accept for many, because it suggests altering some of the deepest traditions and beliefs concerning medical treatment and health. The breakthrough of uncovering conclusive evidence that even life-threatening diseases can be controlled, even wiped out, by the mere willingness to change certain lifestyle choices, threatens the very core of traditional medicine. However, miraculously a few professional medical individuals are joining the ranks, thus helping to position alternative healing as a more acceptable means of healing. Thus, those viewing alternative medicine with criticism may change their views with the backing of a medical field they know and trust.

STEP 7—SEEK OUT OTHERS WHO HAVE BEEN HEALED

The Wellness Center in Clearwater, Florida, keeps a book thick with testimonials of satisfied patients placed on a table near the clinic's entrance.

During my acupuncture treatments, the physicians inquired if I wished to make a testimonial on the success of treatments, which they would publish in their newsletter.

Inquiries can be made to those who have personally experienced certain alternative healing treatments. Most patients are eager to divulge their successful healing experiences and professional healers appreciate this excellent source of advertising of their field. To add most disgruntled patients are very anxious to pass on details of past negative incidents experienced with medical doctors, which initially initiated their interest in seeking into alternative medicine.

Notation

Sharing what you've learned and offering to give testimonies of your experiences, through this type of communication will help develop a substantial alternative healing community and help balance out the powerful controls of the medical establishment. Allow your practitioner to share any information on your healing process with others who are seeking similar care.

STEP 8—FIGHTING FOR THE RIGHT TO BE IN CONTROL

One particular public figure in the past, Senator Strom Thurmond, was responsible for the fight to make nutritional supplements accessible to low-income families. Senator Thurmond had practiced what he preached; celebrating his ninety-fourth birthday on March 9, 1996, he told such dignitaries as former president Nixon, Supreme Court Justice Sandra Day O'Connor, and senators Joseph Biden, Howard Baker, and George Mitchell the following: "Several people here tonight told me that they hoped to come to my 100th birthday party. I told them that if they eat right, take their supplements and keep fit, there is no reason they cannot make it!" Well, the senator did reach his 100th birthday. At that time, a last-minute legislative rider, authored by Senator Orrin Hatch (R- Utah) and strongly supported by Sen. Thurmond, made certain strides in the direction towards the fight for nutritional freedom, which continues sporadically today in the nation's capital. Congressman Bill Richardson (D-NM) sent a letter to his colleagues in the House of Representatives requesting their support of the Dietary Supplement Standards and Consumer Education Act of 1996, which he had planned to introduce that year. In his letter, Rep. Richardson pointed out the role supplements play in promoting good health and prevention of disease, and how an emphasis placed on prevention could reduce America's skyrocketing health care costs.

Thanks to Senator Hatch, Richardson's bill would have similar companion legislation in the Senate. Its intent was to empower consumers to make choices about their own preventive health care programs based on the accurate claims of health benefits related to particular dietary supplements. Jerry Kessler, president of the Nutritional Health Alliance, remarked that aggressive work had to be done to get cosponsors for this legislation and to mobilize grassroots support to ensure its passage.

Unfortunately, while at one time this all looked very promising, nothing has manifested during the Bush administration. History has shown that war devastates the morals of nations in many ways and obliterates peacetime concerns that were once integrated within the societies. In a more harmonious environment, concerns tend to focus more on the proliferation of a higher standard of life, which ideally would include mind, body and spirit, which suggest the developing of humanity's full potentials. There is also greater motivation towards creativity and the arts. In medicine, this creativity could include searching for advanced and more sophisticated means of healing. Obviously, any drastic medical changes depend upon politics, and at present, minimal interest in the advancement of the alternative healing still exists.

Millions of Americans are unable to find relief from chronic ailments from traditional medical care. Chronic fatigue, migraine headaches, back pain, and other common problems, many individuals resign to live with all their lives. Although modern medicine has a realm of specialists, still many ailments, even minor ones, go unresolved. To add, a confusion of contradictions can result from opposing medical specialists' diagnoses, which ultimately leads to a battery of tests. In addition, specialists have a reputation of treating simple ailments as complex emergencies, the "killing a fly with a shotgun" syndrome. On the other hand, alternative healing's focus on cause and effect of illnesses helps to hit the mark more accurately, thus alleviating costly and so often non-effective specialized treatments.

While modern medicine obviously has need for medical specialists, too often this breed is particularly reluctant to see the relationships between various illnesses. An added factor is that specialists are notorious for discounting human emotions playing a role in physical ailments. Tendencies of dissecting patients rather than seeing them as whole, such as the correlations between mind, body and spirit are difficult to grasp.

CHOOSING YOUR DOCTOR

You need to think that if your life was at stake, your doctor would, without question, be your first choice because you trust his method of treatment and that he or she keeps up with the latest healing methods. Most doctors take minimal time reviewing medical journals or the latest medical news. After graduating from medical schools doctors tend to avoid new research, leaving it up to medical scientists.

Depending totally on doctors to heal, results in minimizing responsibility in actively participating in your own healing. Unfortunately, doctors take the attitude that it is entirely their responsibility to heal patients and that patients need only follow their instructions. Like most, my husband's doctor vehemently opposes the validity of alternative healing, to the point of dropping my husband as a patient (similar to my situation), if he persists on seeing an alternative healer. Therefore, the visits to his alternative doctor are kept secret from his primary care physician. The only reason my husband continues to see this doctor is that his insurance covers blood tests and other tests taken in his office, but when any problems pop up, he secretly runs to his alternative doctor for advice. Now the alternative healer in turn is not threatened by my husband's physician and welcomes him because he understands that certain serious medical issues may arise that only his family doctor can address. Nevertheless, the reverse is not the case.

However, gradually my husband depends more on his alternative doctor's advice, and visits him even when not sick, for taking certain preventive treatments such as boosting his immune system to maintain his health. He also was advised to take a regimen of supplements, given nutritional advice, along with a special test for mercury poisoning due to mercury fillings in his mouth. This was followed by a specialized treatment to rid his body of toxic mercury. These treatments would never be available from his doctor.

Making any changes in your healing approach is difficult, for the simple reason that during illness, when patients are most vulnerable, remaining with the familiar offers a sense of comfort. What is even more troublesome is many prior to choosing their doctors, do little investigating regarding their professional attitudes and medical philosophies on healing. The medical board is limited to just offering doctors' medical education, the particular practice they are in and little else.

WORKOUT

Your Health Diary—*Evaluates each question so you can see where you stand with your health. Attempt to understand yourself, regarding your physical well-being.*

1—How would you rate your health…fine, mediocre, or poor? Are there certain times, or under certain conditions, you feel your best or worst?

Perhaps you have settled with not feeling your best or given up attempting to cure some ailment. For example, for some, chronic fatigue is accepted as being normal and perhaps even rationalized it is due to overwork. Chronic fatigue is symptomatic of something wrong in an individual's overall health. This is where alternative healing plays a role. It is does not accept this problem as being normal and thus seeks into its various causes, starting with diet, stress and emotional factors of the patient, and exercise and sleep habits.

2—When you get sick, do you have a difficult time getting well? Explain why you feel you have trouble recovering.

Medical doctors rarely recommend supplements of other preventive care to build up the immune system. Yet the immune system plays a vital role in how rapidly you can recover from illness.

3—Do you attempt to treat yourself of an illness or usually just run to professional care? Explain what self-help healing methods you use.

The usual approach most people take is depending on professionals to heal them, while taking a non-active role in their own health. Each diagnosis received from a doctor should be followed up by intensive research on the whys and wherefores of that particular illness and researching alternative means of addressing such illnesses.

4—Do you get reoccurring illnesses or suffer from chronic problems? Approaching healing as a quick means of feeling better with little regards to actually getting better can progress into a long-term chronichealth condition, since the core of the illness has not be healed.

5—Are you on prescription drugs and are you satisfied with using them?

When physicians prescribe drugs, their side effects are rarely brought up. As far as patients are concerned since they were prescribed by their doctors there should be no questions as to their complete safety. Of course this is not so. Instead medicine is increasingly being questioned as to their safety because of the many serious side effects, some quite deadly. To add, patients have to resort to questioning the pharmacist for such information because the standard attitude from their doctors is the reassurance that the prescribed drug is completely safe. Actually rarely is there a pharmaceutical drug that does not have side effects.

Over-the-counter drugs can be just as harmful for the simple reason that individuals can easily overdose themselves, for example on painkillers, or on the popular painkiller acetaminophen, best known by the Tylenol brand, and which is present in more than 600 products that treat pain, coughs, colds and the flu. Taking these medications on a regular basis can cause liver damage. To make matters worse, many are not aware they are overdosing, and it does not take much to have a negative result. More then 56,000 emergency room visits a year are due to acetaminophen overdoses, where about 100 people a year die after an unintentional overdose of the drug.

This painkiller is not the only culprit. There are other dangerous over-the-counter drugs, such as aspirin, ibuprofen, naproxen, or ketoprofen—called NSAIDs or non-steroidal anti-inflammatory drugs, and side effects include stomach bleeding and kidney problems. Thus, our "friendly pharmacy" does not appear to be so friendly after all. In the meantime, the FDA has neglected its duty by not putting warning labels on these drugs. Again, it is the matter of money, the FDA and drug companies are great financial partners and neither is about to let the other down by complaints made in assuring the public the dangers of the drug world.

6—Do you tend to take your doctor's word as gospel or do you question about certain treatments? You can go to three different doctors and get three different opinions.

7—Have you been searching for a cure for a particular long-term affliction?

Alternative healing offers many healing modalities unavailable in traditional medicine. Medical doctors rarely admit they are not knowledgeable in some areas, thus this can result in patients undergoing scores of tests, and oftentimes with no positive results.

8—Do your friends and family recommend you stay away from untraditional healing methods?

Information on alternative healing is readily accessible at local libraries, health food stores, or on the internet. Once you feel confident in using this type of healing, it will prove difficult for others to talk you out of it. With your acquired knowledge on the subject, you will be able to share your healing experiences with others.

9—Is alternative healing relatively unknown to you? If not, what do you know so far?

Many resolved seeking out traditional medical care because it is so available to them and because usually requires little effort on the part of patients. Alternative healing promotes the concept of self-healing where expectations are patients become more interactive in their healing process.

(Write down how you think you would pursue alternative healing if you were to get sick.)

The following lists ways to find alternative healers and what to look for when selecting an alternative healer.

1—*Word of mouth*—This is the most reliable means of finding a practitioner in your area, particularly if you trust the source.

2—*Search through your reference library*—Some libraries and bookstores offer lectures on alternative healing. For example, if an author has just put out a book on the subject, such as on acupuncture, mind-body healing, pain control—the natural way, etc., now that alternative healing is so widely spread, the reference librarian has access to the information and can provide it to you.

3—*The Internet is a great place to search*—You will not only get general information on health subjects, and national lists of health practitioners that practice in the particular healing field you are looking for, but also a list of practitioners in your area. Make sure to check on their references and testimonials from other patients if you can. They are not always easy to obtain, but with persistence, you will find them. The health clinic I went to had a log jam-packed with handwritten testimonials by pleased patients, placed on a small table where it was readily accessible to new patients. After the treatment, I was asked to write my opinion on my treatment (I always wondered what they do with negative responses).

4—*Seek others in the alternative healing field*—Some healers will make recommendations to other healers, particularly if they are in a different healing field. While practitioners tend to believe they are best in their particular field, however, a massage therapist may recommend acupuncturists, or an herbalist may suggest some homeopathic healer, or natural allergist. In the meantime, those making claims they can heal everything should be avoided. While some practitioners are versatile in their field, rarely is one individual healer an expert in all fields of healing.

5—*Do not be persuaded by negative comments made against alternative healing*— While there are charlatans in every field, too often alternative medicine gets a poor rap. No doubt, mistakes have been made in this field, as in traditional medicine. However, while the latter often gets overlooked, alternative medicine tends to be heavily criticized. There is minimal control over who practices this field; just about anyone can put a sign out front of their place advertising their healing expertise; that is why researching backgrounds are essential.

RADICAL CURES FOR COMMON AILMENTS

KEY WORDS—FOR YOUR JOURNEY TOWARDS NEW WAYS OF HEALING

Trust—While charlatans exist in very field, regarding alternative healing the medical field has denounced it completely. However, while few would refer to failing doctors as charlatans, still thousands of accidental deaths and deadly medical mistakes occurring in hospitals and doctors offices are difficult to understand.

On the other hand, one single incident occurring in the alternative medical field can be disastrous. For example, in the situation with an alternative doctor, David Minkoff, who lost his Florida medical license due to the death of a patient he was treating. No proof was made that any malpractice was involved. It just so happened this doctor was practicing in a field questionable to his accusers who were ready to criticize him at the drop of a hat.

Perseverance—Information on particular alternative healing remedies or practitioners is often not readily available. While the medical field has resources that can help individuals to acquire information such as particular practitioners' backgrounds, no such service is available for alternative healing. Unfortunately, lacking is a centralized system where such information could be available. Due to the nature of this field, where often practitioners find themselves in situations having to defend their practices, rather than developing a cohesive bind with each other, instead a sense of separatism results. This does little to help the movement as a whole or help to assist individuals finding out resources available to them. However, there are ways to get such information. Some alternative practitioners have written books on their particular expertise, or offer lectures, which is an excellent means of learning about various healing modalities used in the alternative healing field and of particular healers. Becoming acquainted with the particular healer you plan to see in the future is good for several reasons; you need to feel this person is compatible to your needs, and also is competent.

Search out reputation—Certain information is available on alternative healing clinics and practitioners, through the licensing bureau, which help to determine if they are licensed, also the department of health of your county, to see if health complaints have been made, Better Business Bureau or the Consumer's Protection Agency to find out if there is any record of complaints against them.

FORGING THROUGH

The number of discontented people with their doctors is growing. Some, realizing the need to be concerned, are demanding to have more control over their health care and thus are questioning the establishment in hopes some alterations can be rendered. Out of this, the Office of Alternative Medicine in the National Institutes of Health has become a reality, and now, available to the public is information on variable health options, and some are even communicating them to their family physicians. Ultimately, this places these doctors in a crunch, because to treat patients they realize the need to keep up with the latest medical data, which some argue includes alternative medicine. To add, it should not be up to patients to inform their doctors that vitamin C helps prevent colds, and acts as a strong antioxidant without being criticized that only an antibiotic drug is beneficial. This is just one of many examples now occurring in doctors' offices across the country.

In any democratic government, free from hierarchical controls, people should have the right not only to choose their doctors but their preferred method of healing. As of now there is only one medical system considered acceptable and dominates health care. However, those fortunate to know of alternative healing methods are aware of their choices, and it is these individuals responsible for initiating possible changes in the system. At the same time, those in the lower income bracket have the least choices, thus, these people are confined to traditional medical care. Because of this, many children at an early age have unnecessarily been on medical drugs most of their lives and often for some minor problems. Usually depending on welfare, sadly, they have little choice.

In the meantime, there are those who realize staying healthy through simple preventive measures is less demanding and less expensive than getting sick.

Insurance companies have not yet figured that one out because if they did, they would promote patients to use alternative medicine to help them from falling into the expenses of getting sick. However, because of the discipline and patience required in many of alternative healing processes, and the tendency to involve a more gradual healing process rather than instant cures, which often are temporary at best, such methods are not appealing to many.

Our ancestors knew well that using certain commonsense means of prevention along with the use of various natural health treatments from the good old-fashioned kitchen stocked with garden herbs was the recipe for good health. However, most of this good sense disappeared with the family herbal gardens, evaporated somewhere in medical test tubes, and trapped within some narrow scope of orthodox medical healing.

Some responsible doctors, troubled by so many discontented and questioning patients, have been forced to reconsider their medical career. Ironically, some are leaving their practices to search into fields of healing unthinkable just a decade ago, and thus becoming involved with alternative medicine in various ways. Some have become practitioners in the field, while others write books, health-wise newsletters, lecture extensively, and even market their own supplements, all of which helps expand the cause. No doubt, changes will be made, and some very unfamiliar healing processes will eventually evolve. For example, perhaps in the future, patients will be instructed by their doctors, rather than "take an aspirin and call me in the morning," to "take a strong multivitamin and you won't need to call me in the morning." A doctor may say, "Take off your clothes," not for an examination, but for a healing massage, done by the nurse, while using some form of "body talk" or visualization process to inform your body to heal itself. While this may appear as some weird medical hocus-pocus at present, this may be the medicine of the future.

CHANGE IS NOT EASY

Medical physicians seeking to add alternative healing to their practice soon discover the vast amount of extra work involved. This includes researching into unfamiliar medical data, which was unavailable in their past traditional training. In a way, it is a re-training in medicine. Suddenly these physicians discover they are not only becoming holistic healers but also constant researchers (a lost art in the medical field, due to the time- consuming factor). For example, time spent on research in maintaining the most current alternative medical data minimizes time for treating patients, which is a steady course of a very profitable income for doctors. Thus, income that is derived from treating the usual number of patients a day, which is about twenty-five, with each patient receiving less than fifteen minutes with the doctor, affects the very financial business of the physician's office practice. Very few doctors are willing to give up a lucrative medical practice to venture into something unfamiliar, where perhaps monetary rewards are questionable.

This is the basic reason why many chiropractors and D.O. are more open to alternative medicine. For one thing, chiropractors do not administer medicine, and thus have turned their attention towards other healing methods. For example, some focus on the concept that the spinal column controls health and a spine out of alignment results in various physical problems, some that may appear completely disconnected to any chiropractic problems. Acupuncture and massage, both included in alternative healing, have been steadily added to chiropractic practice, the particular benefit being they are often covered by health insurance. Unfortunately, in the past, chiropractors have acquired shady reputations, mostly due to medical doctors disclaiming their validity. Unfortunately, the refusal of the University of South Florida's acceptance of a chiropractic education division, for the simple reason that this form of healing is considered questionable by traditional medicine, did not help them in acquiring a stamp of validity.

Hopefully, in the future, doctors will take note of their patients who have experienced some form of natural healing and perhaps learn from them.

Actually, very few have not heard something about alternative healing since information is so available, but in turn, the medical establishment still remains sequestered from it. It is very difficult for doctors to refrain from prescribing drugs for every illness to the point that given even a hint of infection an antibiotic is often automatically prescribed. Recently, the news media gave a report that doctors are unnecessarily prescribing too much antibiotics. For example, when a patient is suffering from sore throat, rather than going through the normal procedure of taking a strep throat test, doctors not wishing to take up this time, just issue an antibiotic. The problem is after a while patients become immune to antibiotics, thus, if a major infection should strike an effective defense is jeopardized…

In the meantime, many infections and viruses such as the flu, sinus problems, even colds are effectively healed by such means as herbs; echinacea and goldenseal, vitamin C, elderberry and zinc, and none require paying doctors' fees or prescriptions. Even better, these remedies help the body to heal itself rather than temporarily patch up the illnesses.

While medical doctors are notorious for not budging from medical data learned in their education, those in alternative healing are constantly learning innovative ways of healing as new research in this field becomes available. For example, numerous doctors practice chelation therapy; however, research came up with a new approach in this area. The standard sodium EDTA which most chelation therapists use requires a three-hour treatment, which is a long time for some patients to sit. Now some chelation doctors are offering a "fast-track" calcium EDTA chelation that can be done in a few minutes. Since initially venturing in the long journey of collecting information for this book, numerous modalities have evolved. For example, various therapies regarding sound, psychic, spiritual and hands-on healing, while existing for some time, have expanded in many new directions and expectations are that more will become manifested in the future.

A study made by Dr. Emanuel Cheraskin, professor emeritus at the University of Alabama Medical School, who published more then 460 medical papers and has some 210 citations to his credit, for the National Library of Medicine decided to find a large group of healthy people and see what nutrients they were consuming, and in what amounts. He mailed two nationally recognized survey forms, the Cornell Medical Index and the Standard Food Frequency Questionnaire, to several thousand dentists and their families. The Cornell form obtains very personal health information including subtle, often overlooked symptoms of illness such as aches, pains, colds and allergies. Not surprisingly, the people in the survey with the highest nutrient intake were the healthiest and those taking the fewest suffered more symptoms of illness. Conversely, Dr. Cheraskin found the fewer nutrients that were ingested, the more prevalent were the nagging symptoms of ill health. However, what was surprising was that the healthiest people were exceeding the government's minimal RDA's (recommended dietary allowance) for vitamins and minerals by five to ten times. Now take this data to your doctor next time he or she writes out a prescription for you.

CHAPTER 5

CHANGING UNHEALTHY HABITS

We are a nation bred on junk food, often referred to as "dead food," lacking fiber and enzymes, and deficient in proper vitamins and minerals. Surprisingly, very few regard nutrition as the most important part of the pillar of good human health. It has been only in the past few decades that nutrition and its role in health have come to the forefront. Unfortunately, while most individuals are aware of the relationship between nutrition and health, often this vital subject is ignored, basically because we have become a people who have lost the sense of moderation and discipline, which are required to maintain good health.

The human body, as a complex organism, has the amazing ability to heal itself; however, you must make certain efforts for this to apply. Whether through exposure to environmental toxins, poor nutrition, cigarette smoking, alcohol consumption, or inactivity, our bodies endure much abuse. Still it can usually serve us for us many years before starting to break down. The body is composed of millions of little engines, some working in unison, some working independently, but all working on-call twenty-four hours a day. However, for these engines to work at full capacity, specific fuels are required. Unfortunately, if this fuel is the wrong blend, the engine will run poorly.

The body's fuel determines its level of ability to function at its full capacity at present and in the future. Unfortunately, certain bodily dysfunctions can be difficult to detect in their early stages, thus subtle but vital health issues can go unnoticed. A health problem can be so obscure that it goes undetected for years and then only to manifest itself when we age or grow weak for some reason. This is particularly evident with the growth of cancer. This disease can be so insidious and hidden that it is easy for it to go undetected for years. In addition, diabetes is another disease that can go undetected for years until it becomes a full-blown problem, which then is usually too late to take measures to prevent it.

Alternative healing focuses on the prevention of disease, and detecting those diseases before they grow and become a major problem. That means the immune system needs to work at full capacity by keeping it well nourished and the body physically strong. Very few are fortunate enough to be so healthy that abusive eating habits will not eventually have an effect on their health. Although we are living longer, and many modern medical advantages are available, still medical reports claim Americans are not the healthiest of people. Actually, in the past decade it shows Americans suffer from more ailments than did their ancestors, although there are more medical opportunities available to them.

EAT WHAT GROWS AROUND YOU AND WHEN IT IS IN SEASON

The ancient Oriental adage "Eat what grows around you and when it is in season" was a rule followed in order to determine the most nutritional foods. Most of us do not live in a Garden of Eden environment, so our only foods, from soil, are usually located a distance from us. Our ancestors consumed live foods that way in their immediate surrounding, fresh from the garden or directly from the hunt. Evolving from the primate species, where food sources derived directly from nature, ideally that should be our source of food. However, today foods come far from the sources in which they originated, and consequently are rarely consumed when in their prime maturity; either they are over- ripened or not ripen enough. To add, through preserving, processing and undergoing periods of ripening, by the time they reach the table nothing much is left of the foods' natural nutrition. Through the development of various process technologies, foods can be picked months before consumption and in that time ultimately evolve into food completely devoid of any nutritional value.

Since today's food is produced primarily for profit, health concerns are often sacrificed. Vegetables and fruits are grown in soils depleted from pesticides, a toxin formulated to kill over 150 species of insects. Farmers drench the soil with these toxins, thus robbing it of its natural nutrients, in turn producing weakened plants drained of vitamins and minerals. Rarely, in today's fast-paced world is produce ripened naturally on the vine where it can reach its full nutritional maturity. Fruits and vegetables are picked unripe to prevent spoiling before they reach the market. Often while appearing healthy and ripe, nutritional value is depleted from the unripe shipping. Nutritionists recommend that all produce be consumed within three days from when it was picked, which is almost impossible. First required is the time to harvest, then transporting to destinations sometimes thousands of miles away, followed by sitting in grocery stores until eventually purchased and then sitting in the fridge until time to use. To add, some means of transportation goes unrefrigerated (the best means of keeping produce fresh), particularly produce imported from warmer climates, such as from Central and South America. So in order to utilize all this produce much goes through a chain of food processing such as canning, freezing and drying, which destroys fresh nutrients. As the nutritionist and alternative medical doctor Jay Rown, MD, says, a good rule to follow is "If God did not make it, think twice before consuming it, and only consume food the way nature intended."

Most nutritionists agree that many food sources should be consumed raw. Our prehistoric ancestors only cooked meat and ate all vegetables and fruit raw. Another good rule to follow is the more colorful the food, the healthier it likely is, and foods with crisp textures offer more fiber than soft food. A study showed that the pancreas of rats enlarges due to the increased demand for digestive enzymes when they were fed processed foods lacking enzymes. This resulted in eventually exhausting the ability of the pancreas to make digestive enzymes, thus individuals or animals suffer further damage from poor nutrition. Sprouted grains and legumes because their vitamins and minerals have been released at the plant's budding age are considered very nutritious. At the same time, the carbohydrate portion of milled grain is largely devoid of food value. To add, by testing on random vegetables taken off the shelf, scientists discovered that organic foods contained significantly more vitamins and minerals than commercial vegetables and lacked the dangerous pesticide toxins. Since so much fast food is deep-fried in saturated oils, thus causing cholesterol problems (a growing epidemic with young people), the question is what are the most suitable cooking oils? The answer is narrowed down to two, and those are organic extra-virgin olive oil and coconut oil. However, fast food and other restaurants, as well as school cafeterias, do not use these oils for the simple reason they are more expensive. To add, cooking oils sold in plastic bottles are best to avoid because oil is a solvent petrochemical and plastics are made from petrochemicals; to make it flexible highly toxic phthalates are added. They can easily leach out right into the oil used in cooking, since they are oil soluble. The bottom line is that phthalates are injurious to body organs and should be avoided whenever possible.

ORGANIC FOODS

Unfortunately, organic foods are out of reach, price wise, for many. Even more frustrating, health stores selling organic foods are rare. For many, health stores are considered a luxury, even though the food they carry is safer and more nutritional than that available in the average American supermarket. Several years ago, organic produce was less than desirable, at least visually, and variety was scarce. Fruits appeared overly ripe and covered with brown spots, and leafy vegetables were sadly wilted. That has changed; now organic produce can easily be compare, both visually and in variety, to non-organic produce, and of course, the organic is far superior to the inorganic.

Many organic farms have sprouted throughout the states, though most are concentrated in California and have grown into profitable businesses. No longer delegated to small out-of-reach plots of land owned by dedicated altruistic farmers who usually were far from successful, organic produce has grown into big business. Publics, far removed from anything close to health foods or organic produce, have finally joined the bandwagon and carry a limited supply of organic produce. Also on their shelves are an assortment of soy products, but still they have a far way to go. Until customers make demands for healthier foods and where it becomes affordable this supermarket's supply will remain meager. At our present stage, such change is unlikely because the average American diet has grown worse in the past several years despite increasing information and resources regarding diet and health. Thus, this indicates a gap between knowing about good eating habits and making the effort to do so.

HEALTH AND POOR EATING HABITS (WE ARE WHAT WE EAT)

Malnutrition and its various forms can begin as early as childhood, even though the body is receiving plenty of food. Often, those who are overweight suffer from lack of proper nutrients, thus, resulting in the overeating syndrome because improper food has been consumed. Nutrition lists claim the acronym for the "standard American diet" is SAD. Brought up on convenient, prepackaged "substances" which are largely lacking nutritional substances and provide only empty calories, more children suffer obesity, largely because they consume large amounts of fattening food to make up for the lack of eating nutritional food. For example, just one soft drink per day (totally devoid of nutrition), is full of calories and also doubles a child's risk of obesity and childhood diabetes. To add, American's most popular menu, hamburger and fries, loaded with fat and calories, has minimal food value. Yet many children survive on this menu and little else for the simple reason they are readily available just about everywhere. Sadly, while poor diets are often the cause of heart disease, high cholesterol, and diabetes, which is well known through the United States, these bad eating habits are ignored by the medical establishment; compounded by family doctors avoiding informing patients of the cause and effect of dysfunctional lifestyles and health; this only adds to the problem.

Many years ago, the renowned Westin Price traveled the world visiting aboriginal communities to determine the basis for these peoples' tremendous good health.

Price found that groups untouched by civilization and living only by primitive means compared to our standards experienced robust health with minimal degenerative disease, only one dental cavity per 100 teeth, no need for braces, and well-balanced mental health. It was concluded that the consumption of their native and natural diet was the cause of their fine health. The situation is similar in other more primitive societies. When left alone by the outside world, minimal health problems existed, but when visited by foreign civilizations that introduced their diets and ways of life, diseases of all kinds engulfed the inhabitants.

Remaining healthy requires dedication and discipline. One of the most obvious health factors is obesity because it carries with it so many problems. Fortunately, controlling this problem depends upon individuals making the right choice, where illnesses from poor eating habits can be avoided. One troublesome health factor is that poor health habits may not manifest themselves until years later in people's lives. However, increasingly at the present time, younger people are suffering from old-age diseases and pediatricians report an alarming rate of kids suffering from diabetes and cholesterol problems. Many forty-year-olds are suffering from a variety of diseases unheard of with this age group in the past.

To add, poor eating habits do not always indicate being overweight. Individuals can be thin and still be unhealthy, and oftentimes suffer from anemia or burn off energy from perhaps a nervous disorder. Surely, such conditions are far from healthy. While the increase of a diversity of exercising programs, in-vogue memberships to spas, gyms, personal trainers, this trend usually does not include learning about good eating habits. Individuals can go on diets to lose weight but still be on a poor diet. In our rushed, stressful world, junk food is too plentiful and easily obtainable, making it a tempting curse to indulge. Of course, TV food commercials do not help; they can be considered one major culprit in feeding viewers well-designed colorful advertisement of one junk food or another. Overeating or having poor health habits renders one more vulnerable to all sorts maladies for the simple reason that having less self- control can lead to any form of addiction. Having a sense of control and being charge over one's own health and lifestyle by adherence to certain simple rules regardless of external influences promotes a sense of wellness that is priceless.

CHAPTER 6

ENVIRONMENTAL POLLUTION AND HEALTH

This subject could fill volumes. Research shows that we are more exposed to contaminated chemicals than previously thought. Before the industrial revolution, we ate food in an environment containing only naturally occurring compounds and elements that sustained life. The last fifty years have seen an explosion of new manmade chemicals. Today at least 30,000 chemicals never before seen on the planet are mass-produced and released into the environment. We are digging up the earth and releasing literally thousands of naturally occurring heavy metals that Mother Nature had safely tucked away within the innards of the planet. Eventually they make their way into the food chain. We are simultaneously adding a multitude of chemicals called preservatives into our foods. Some of these foods are artificial substances that the human body was never intended to consume. It is no wonder cancer has become an epidemic in our country.

An increasing number of substances are being added to the list of potentially harmful environmental pollutants. Unfortunately, since determining exactly what is harmful to the health of humans is difficult, many of these toxins go unnoticed and therefore untreated. It does not help that the medical field is in denial as to the effects of environmental pollutants. Doctors' unwillingness to recognize a substance as harmful is dependent upon them seeing evidence that the agent directly produces ill effects. Conventional laboratory tests are too gross to measure subtle abnormalities like those produced by food allergies and sensitivities to other common environmental agents. Thus, developing a more sensitive testing system that will detect the effects of chemicals on the physical body after consuming these foods laden with additives, and our exposure to environmental chemicals is essential in determining the health of future generations.

Conventional medicine fails to observe the many unseen subtle influences affecting health. Environmental illnesses relating to exposure to toxic substances levels are levels higher than FDA safety limits. The inability of conventional scientific testing to measure subtle negative disturbances to human physiology certainly limits the FDA's ability to define exactly which substances are truly detrimental to the human body, let alone the precise concentration necessary for toxic effects.

An interesting case in point is how the toxic factors of common household utensils go undetected. For example, the inexpensive cooking aluminum pot may release a possible toxin that may damage our brains. When the aluminum pots or pans are scrubbed or stirred while cooking or washing, infinitesimally small amounts of aluminum metal are dissolved, released, and unknowingly consumed. Recent findings suggest that even larger amounts of aluminum are released, particularly if fluoridated water is used. Food stored in aluminum cans may also contain toxins leached out of the metal. Tests show this type of subtle aluminum toxin absorption, as well the introduction of other environmental toxins, can have a detrimental effect on the brain cells. Some recent research involving Alzheimer's disease, an increasing cause of dementia in the population, has shown that a significant number of patients with this disorder have high aluminum levels in their brain tissue.

There are many substances in our environment including asbestos, PCB's, dioxin and formaldehyde, which orthodox scientists have only begun to acknowledge as harmful or stressful to human beings, and many more are still unknown to scientists. In the meantime, the ability to define chemical stress to the human system depends upon the sensitivity of the measurement systems used to detect both detrimental chemicals and their effects on the welfare of humans.

Some alternative physicians use certain types of sensitive testing on their patients to detect subtle disarrangements in the body; traditional medical doctors do not recognize these tests because these minute irregularities are too insignificant for them to be concerned. However, such subtleties revealing that something is not quite right in the body can potentially help to prevent major illnesses developing. This is the role alternative healing is about; it focuses on prevention of ailments before they can expand into serious diseases. In addition, there are methods to help release toxins in the body, again, which help to prevent future medical problems. Seeking various subtle misalignments in the human system often can prevent such diseases as Alzheimer, Parkinson, and other degenerative disorders. In an environment inundated with many variable pollutants (many were nonexisting a few years ago), causes of the epidemic growth of cancers still remains perplexing. Therefore, taking preventive measures in detecting medical irregularities existing in their earliest stage helps minimizes the risk of them manifesting into full problems.

THE PERILS OF PESTICIDES

Again, we cannot say enough about the issue of pesticides in our food system. Perhaps the worst offenders are the vast array of pesticides now easily obtainable by the average consumer, who uses them in abundance in nearly every American household. Obviously, the most manicured lawns use the most pesticides in order to maintain that perfect bright green so prevalent in golf courses.

Then this tendency to overuse pesticides spreads to our food system. Even the most efficient homemaker rarely considers the pesticide residue left on fruits and vegetables, instead relying on the supermarket to sell healthy foods. Unfortunately, most food products miss the mark. While our market fruits and vegetables may appear on the surface to be attractive, they can be akin to the perfectly bright, delicious-looking red but poisonous apple as told in a fairy tale.

Glorified as saviors of food production, pesticides cause all sorts of problems including cancer, neurological degeneration, and diseases we do not yet know of. For example, analysis of breast tumors can unearth a significant amount of various toxins consumed by the individual. They may be stored away for years in the fatty tissues of the breast, right up against very sensitive mammary tissues that are vulnerable to cancerous degeneration.

We cannot say enough about pesticides and insecticides. Laboratory tests have shown that such toxins interfere with the nervous systems of animals. Common sense should tell us that anything that kills, even if the victim is as tiny as an insect, must have toxic properties. The gradual buildup of ingesting these toxins in our system, which is evident in our commercial food chain, will result in negative consequences.

Scientists in Alaska were baffled at the presence of pesticide residues found in a wilderness lake, where just a few years earlier none was apparent. The lake is located far from any human environment or where the local people had used the pesticide, thus, it was concluded that this toxin had traveled a long distance. Studies further showed that otters of the Columbia River are sterile, with mixed external genitals, and the Florida Everglades alligators are losing their ability to reproduce. Sciences point to pesticides, in parts per trillion, being capable of exerting direct toxicity on the immature Alpha and reproductive organs of the animals, causing improper sexual functions and mixed nonfunctioning genitals. These chemicals seem to exert an effect far more powerful than commonly realized. It would require more than a volume to report all the researchers that have proven how deadly toxins are to the human system.

To make matters worse, researchers have shown through tests that certain pests are becoming resistant and more highly toxic chemicals have to be used to control or kill them. In the meantime, it has been proved that if plants are grown in nutrient-rich soil that is comprised mainly of natural manure and well taken care of, they grow an inner strength that can actually ward off disease and insects. However, all this requires time and care, and nurturing plants for mass commodity and profit is what farming is all about. The massive production of food products has become a profit-making industry, which unfortunately takes minimal responsibility for the safety of its products.

Along with others, I have been protesting the use of pesticides, which has reached epidemic proportions in Florida due to the expansive green spaces of the many golf courses and parklands. Despite copious research on the detrimental effect of pesticide use in relation to human health factors, still turf and trees are incessantly sprayed within human habitat areas, and even more detrimental around water edges to control growth where cutting lawn trackers are unable to reach. Environmentalists claim this fungicide-pesticide not only kills this growth but the many life forms living there and destroys nesting areas for turtles and various aquatic birds. To add, when it rains, this toxic residue runs into the water, thus polluting it, which is detrimental to wildlife and birds whose drinking sources are these water areas. Aquatic birds are hit the hardest since their survival depends upon the waters for a safe and healthy food supply. Since water collects and holds toxins, these feeding areas are polluted and the birds become endangered.

TESTIMONY

I personally observed a dove that made a nest in one of my old flowerpots, laid some eggs, and consistently sat on them for several days. Suddenly, she left, never to return. Gradually the eggs started to turn gray and I then discovered they were infertile. Doves eat grass seed found on lawns, and our neighborhood lawns are inundated with pesticides. I believe this to be largely responsible for those infertile eggs. I suppose toxins of one sort or another are causing this problem all over our planet, but the importance of the situation hit me fully when I observed the damage firsthand, though perhaps in a minuscule way.

    A similar incident involving a medical doctor's experience with her daughter's terrible miscarriage further convinced me of my theory. Upon coming to the United States, Dr. Felicia Spuza opened a medical clinic, and when her son and daughter graduated from medical school in Romania, they joined her. They all were heavily into pharmaceutical drugs. The mother, whom I became friends with, seemed to have become victim of every drug salesman that entered through her door. When visiting her one day, I was taken aback by the powerful medicinal odor fumigating her office and told her about it. I suppose she listened because, after a time, her office gradually smelled less like a pharmaceutical factory and apparently, she took notice of them because the door to the clinic was often left opened. However, as for her daughter's miscarriage, I believe the heavy usage of pharmaceutical drugs played an integral part.

Perhaps the most poisonous widely disseminated substance around is fluoride, which is deliberately added to drinking water, supposedly to reduce tooth decay, though this has never been proven. It has been proven, however, that fluoride can wreck havoc on the DNA repair enzyme, the destruction of which can result in severe cellular disruption or even cancer. Yet there is not a dentist that does not offer fluoride treatments, along with another unhealthy dental care, specifically mercury fillings. Even though by now much evidence has been revealed of the detrimental health factors of mercury fillings, dentists are still using them. What makes it so sad is that children unable to afford non-mercury fillings, which can be expensive, are being placed in such unhealthy situations.

PLASTIC POISON

Then there are plastics, which are themselves a class of chemical compounds. This substance is virtually found in just about every frozen food product. Actually plastic wraps of one kind or another are so common that it would be rare to find a household that did not have this product. The plasticizers are used to make plastic soft, so it is able to wrap around our foods to keep them fresh. The problem is that these toxic compounds leak into our foods and drinks. They are one of the most insidious classes of compounds, which have found their way into our food sources, damaging the liver, kidneys, and especially the reproductive organs.

PERILS OF ELECTROMAGNETIC FIELDS

Electrical magnetic pollution can be caused even by low-energy electromagnetic fields. Living near high-tension power lines, radio or television transmitters, and other appliances that give off such energy may all contribute to health problems. Even access to cellular phones or working in front of video display terminals can be hazardous. Biological systems have been shown to be sensitive to such energy, and react by growing cancer cells. Conflicts regarding this subject are perpetuated by those in the industry and energy fields, who have a vested interest in proving these sources do not produce harm, just as those in the chemical industry must promise and improve the safety of pesticides.

However, this hotly debated topic is far from being settled. The so-called "icing on the cake" in food preservation is any form of radiation, which is overtly damaging to the body's molecules, yet much of our food supply is being bombarded with radiation in an effort to get that longer shelf life. The radiation is so forceful that it smashes apart chemical bonds, freeing atoms to reunite in unnatural ways and create molecules called radial lights, compounds never before seen on the planet. Do you think our immune systems would know what to do with strange unnatural transformations? The only safe conclusion here is to avoid irradiated food at all cost.

MERCURY POISON

Few people are aware of mercury poison, a possibility for those with fillings in their teeth. Many dentists still use mercury, though some have begun using other, safer methods for cavity work. The question is, how can you detect whether you have mercury poison, or any other heavy metals in your system, and then be rid of them? To detect mercury toxins some natural practitioners do a hair analysis. This method is not approved or recognized by the FDA, because an individual needs to have a heavy case of this toxin in their system before it's legally deemed unsafe. Unfortunately, usually at this governmentally mandated level, the damage caused by toxic metals has already occurred. Alternative physicians remove mercury from the body through DMPS IV's along with oral chelation. To start, a urine analysis is taken to detect the level of toxins. Then, DMPS puts the metals into the bloodstream and oral chelation moves it from the blood into the urine. After several treatments, another urine analysis is taken to see if all toxins are vacated.

LEAD POISON

In recent years, the EPA has estimated that modern humans have up to 700 times more lead in their bones than did our ancestors. We have been exposed to high doses of lead in gasoline, which adds to the other set of high levels of heavy metals in the environment. By now, most of us are aware of the stories regarding little children who eat old paint from chipped windowsills...that is LEAD paint. The public demanded that this unnecessary toxin be removed from their homes, and now house paint no longer contains lead. However, there are still many insidious ways lead can creep into the system. According to some alternative specialists, lead poisoning is so prevalent that they claim many common ailments are the result of just a small amount of lead in an individual's system. Unfortunately, the average blood test does not usually detect small amounts of this destructive toxin and thus special tests are required, and usually not covered by any insurance.

The question is who defines where heavy metal poisoning begins? Your vascular disease symptoms are a much better predictor of heavy metal poisoning than commonly accepted lab numbers. There was a time when "authorities" told us certain levels of lead were "safe" and did not have any known side effects. For example, at one time medical officials diagnosed lead poisoning if blood levels were above 60 mcg per deciliter (mcg/dl), a level that is high enough to result in kidney injury, serious abdominal problems, and severe brain damage. Following studies in the

1980s and '90s, the allowable level was reduced by the Centers for Disease Control (CDC) to 30 mcg/dl in 1975, 25 mcg/dl in 1985, and to the current level of 10 mcg/dl in 1991. (This last figure correlates to 100 parts per billion.)

Lead poisoning is so prevalent that there is belief that vascular disease is one of the first symptoms the body exhibits, sexual dysfunction following closely behind. Sadly, only a small amount of lead in the system can cause such problems, though it easily can go undetected. Recent discoveries indicate that lead poisoning actually occurs at a fraction of the current definably toxic level, and is believed to be the cause of various health problems, including sexual dysfunction, mental disease, hypertension and various forms of heart disease. A study recently published in the *New England Journal of Medicine* reported that children's IQs fall by some 4.6 points for every 10 mcg/dl rise in lead level above the supposedly safe level of 10 mcg/dl. Further research showed that extremely low levels, only 1 mcg/dl, affected a child's IQ. Ultimately, it was discovered that the IQ declined by 7.4 points as lifetime average blood lead concentrations increased from 1 to 10 mcg/dl.

Understanding how just a minuscule amount of lead has devastating negative effects on children, think how you have been harboring lead a lot longer than children have, and consequently it is rational why hormonal and sexual dysfunction in adults is even more apparent. Most of today's adults grew up in an era when so-called "safe" levels of lead were significantly higher than they are today, and there is an increased chance they have proportionally more lead in their systems because caution to stay away from lead sources was much less adamant.

A report made by the prestigious *Journal of the American Medical Association* (*JAMA*) headed by Denis Nash, PhD, and his team at the University of Maryland followed 2,165 women age 40 to 59 years. The article reported the team's findings and summarized the findings of other lead studies. Their results were compelling. No doubt, there was a direct connection between lead and hypertension in rats and other animals, and now it was proven for humans as well. Evidence showed that lead in the body resulted in erratic behavior patterns, electrical rhythm disturbances of the heart, abnormal pumping function, abnormal vascular muscle tissue, and direct action on parts of the nervous system responsible for blood pressure regulation.

Men with hypertension have significantly higher levels of lead in their system than normal, reports a 1996 *JAMA* article, and "cumulative lead exposure." Moreover, it does not take much lead to do its negative job. *JAMA* suggests that the smallest amount of lead in one's system is dangerous, and that because of this testing for lead poison should become customary, as is checking a patient's blood pressure, cholesterol, and the possibility of diabetes. Dr. Richard Canfield of Cornell University, one of the *JAMA* study's lead authors, emphatically stated, "The fact is, in our study, we found no evidence for a safe level of exposure."

Blood tests cannot accurately detect lead in the system. A challenge specimen utilizing a chelating agent such as EDTA is a more accurate means to mobilize lead from bone stores. For thirty-five years, traditional medicine has vehemently attempted to eliminate the practice of chelation. Oral chelation should be a vital part of one's daily supplement regimen. Because it is most likely that just about every individual has some amount of lead in their system, particularly seniors and those from the baby boom generation who have had many years to collect this poison, everyone should go on a daily dose of oral chelation. This means adding a product providing calcium EDTA, at least four grams per day for an average-sized adult, to your daily health routine. Garlic also chelates lead and zinc; calcium protects enzymes against lead toxicity. However, you need a broad-spectrum mineral supplement to replace nutritional minerals that might be removed from EDTA. To enhance this treatment, a regular dose of the fast-push calcium EDTA to get higher blood levels of the chelator and deeper penetration is recommended.

The American Board of Chelation Therapy is expanding in many directions and changing its horizons. It is now called the American Board of Clinical Metal Toxicology, and personnel can be reached at 800-356-2228. The number of doctors using chelation on their patients is increasing. However, unless insurance companies determine that a patient's lead level is high enough, which means dangerously high, chelation expenses are not covered. Furthermore, the latest research published in some very prestigious medical journals may encourage many to consider the need for heavy metals blood test. Given the information on the dangers of the minutest bit of lead in the system, everyone should qualify for a formal diagnosis of lead poisoning and insurance reimbursement. It may require some persistence, but insurance companies should cover both the test and the treatment. These preventive tests are important yet are rarely included in regular medical exams. Tending to wait until an illness is obvious and well settled in the human system, the medical field pays minimal attention to taking preventive measures. They have yet to accept that such practice curtails serious future health problems. Treating small problems before they expand and become complicated is much more productive; do not wait until the damage is done.

From birth, most of us have been provided with a wondrous immune system, and all we have to do is carefully maintain our inner healing forces. Nature intended us to fuel these mechanisms with the right natural substances to enable the body to function to its full capacity. Our immune systems are designed to keep us healthy even when struggling with diverse conditions. However, with the many toxins that exist within the environment, this wonderful immune system is often challenged. While at the mercy of multitudinous toxins, rejuvenating certain damages can be achieved through various alternative healing modalities.

WORKOUT

Follow these steps to avoid and rid yourself of toxins:

1—Find a reliable source where you can be tested for toxins and go through a detox program.

2—Avoid mercury fillings and aluminum sources (cookware and canned foods).

3—Avoid settling for the broad or vague tests offered by most physicians, which do not detect subtle toxins in the system.

4—Maintain your knowledge of natural health and healing through written materials such as books and research work available on the Internet.

5—Look into some common supplements that are good detoxing agents, such as vitamins C and E.

6—Include in your diet plenty of organic, raw fruits and vegetables.

7—Try to use natural materials wherever you can.

CHAPTER 7

EMBRACING THE OLD WITH THE NEW

THE HUMAN BODY IS NOT A MACHINE

In earlier times in the medical science field, the understanding of human structure and function was limited. The human body was often likened to an intricate machine made up of pumps, pistons, gears, and pulleys and which was projected within the culture of the times. For example, in the art media, the early-twentieth-century paintings by the French artist Ferdinand Leger depicted female figures as abstract pieces of machinery. His paintings consisted of female legs and arms as bright enamel-painted metal tubing and other body parts as metal shields. These figures represented the coming of the machine age of the turn of the nineteenth century, with the development and implementation of engines. However, as in most offensive trends, there were those who questioned the disruption of the status quo and criticized this movement simply because it was believed machines would eventually replace human labor.

Such an analogy can be somewhat compared to current medical attitudes in their tendency to take a dehumanizing approach towards treating patients. The complaint made against the current medical paradigm, usually by those practicing alternative medicine, is that too often patients are treated as mere body parts, their illnesses channeled into certain categories. If a patient suffers a problem outside of these categories, then chances are it will be untreatable. The tendency towards dehumanization approaches in orthodox medicine and how the body is viewed as being made up of separate parts, almost machine like, is exemplified by the physician's common view that the heart is merely a physical engine of strength and precision. Simplistically, they have attempted to duplicate its function through the creation of the artificial heart. Many problems have evolved from attempts to replace the human heart with an artificial one, such as reoccurring strokes and subsequent neurological problems.

While medical doctors have their explanation for this problem, another analysis has been considered, though questionable by the medical establishment. It is believed the heart chakra (an ancient concept) supplies the physical heart with nutritive etheric energy, which may be the higher energetic source of dysfunction contributing to the degeneration of the heart. It is interesting to note that dysfunction of the heart chakra due to emotional blockages involving the expression of love to oneself and others is not associated with physical diseases of the heart, including coronary artery disease, various cardiomyopathies, and strokes related to stasis of circulation. Perhaps the ailing heart chakra of mechanical heart transplant recipients is the overriding subtle energy factor that causes recurrent strokes, and not any physical defects within the device. Thus, this would suggest that those with an actual human heart transplant might be able to live comfortably with their new heart if willing to undergo various alternative healing modalities, such as chakra meditation, intended to touch upon the emotional aspect of the heart.

This concept can extend into dealing with other ailments. For example, those suffering from chronic headaches and other disturbances due to stress could focus on the crown chakra for healing. This includes meditation on the area on top of the head where a lotus flower opening up in bloom is envisioned. Those with eye problems, particularly individuals having myopic vision, perhaps may be suffering from a social disorder, such as being over critical and non-receptive. (In essence, we see what we wish to see and hear what we wish to hear.) This chakra healing, an ancient healing practice from India, is done by meditating on the back of the head, behind the eyes, at one of the chakra points.

In addition, respiratory ailments of any kind, including chronic sinus ailments and sore throats, can be the result of how the voice is used, such as emoting stressful or angry harsh tones, which puts a stress on the throat. The throat chakra, another chakra point, located behind the throat in the neck area, in the healing process is visualized as the sipping a cool fruit beverage.

In conclusion, since we are not made of just mere body parts, our senses and bodily organs are aligned with a multitude of external conditions, and are affected in a myriad of ways other than what appears simplistically obvious. Alternative healing regards illness as more complex than traditional medicine views it and often existing beyond common medical knowledge. Thus, causes of illnesses are viewed as endless and oftentimes existing with their own rhyme and reason. When patients are treated in a fragmented manner, that is where the totality of a complete human being is not recognized in any kind of healing treatment, mind, body, spirit; mechanically dissecting illnesses, measuring them in test tubes, robs the very essence of the meaning of healing. There are too many layers of the human consciousness that are imbedded within a patient's psyche that need consideration in any given medical treatment. Thus traditional medicine does little integrating of an individual's spiritual and emotional well-being, and considers them separate issues, as they do with individual illnesses. Disregarding the connection between the mind, body and spirit in any given illness is a disservice to patients because the deeper layers of potential causes of illnesses go unheeded.

Suffering from severe chronic illnesses, perhaps to the point of sequestering the patient from their former positions in life, can be a depressing experience, particularly for those who were active participators in the community. Thus, self-esteem and one's sense of dignity can be threatened, resulting in lack of interest in activities and separation from friends and family. Alternative healing takes such factors into consideration when dealing with patients. It realizes healing encompasses more than physical concerns. Going beyond the boundaries of doctors and medicine, it attempts to encompass the realm of humanistic concerns, which includes the whole human being—mind, body and spirit.

HEALING IN ANCIENT ATLANTIS

The story of Atlantis serves as an appropriate introduction to what may be considered by some as exotic and even difficult to believe, and that is the art of healing with the use of crystals. Atlanteans were able to detect many of the principles of directing crystalline energies for the purpose of healing. This included the manipulation of subtle energies and knowledge of the connection between the physical and subtle bodies. Today's interest in the healing powers of crystals echoes the crystal power so evident in a civilization existing several thousand years ago. Actually, historians are able to find some of this ancient data regarding crystal healing, but the present gap between the medical world and such discoveries will curtail much of this information ever reaching the medical field. This is because crystal healing does not fit into the modern "test tube" medical mentality. While we may have our hands on such wondrous knowledge, there is little chance of utilizing any of it, at least for the present time.

To add to this mysticism surrounding the healing arts of the ancient races, a recent archeological excavation in Egypt near the Sphinx and the Great Pyramid was led by the famous psychic healer Edgar Cayce and his foundation, along with a team from Stanford University and the Egyptian government. This excavation site was chosen due to the psychic information derived from Cayce's readings, which gave information on a certain tunnel that led to the Pyramid of Records. This location was believed to contain a time capsule having a record of the healing powers of crystals from Atlantis.

ANCIENT HEALING WITH LIGHT

The timeless healing practice existing in the ancient lost continent Atlantis involved healing power of light and color. This culture knew of the pranic forces carried by sunlight, which was believed to be the subtle energetic significance to all living cells. Powerful healing forces of color produced by the sunlight passing through crystalline prisms, as well as the healing octave color rays were also studied. Over centuries, the Atlanteans' rise to a high state of technological achievement enabled them to tap into and use the sun's energy for creation and sustenance in their society. The sun, regarded as a healer and worshipped as a god, was the very essence of these people's lives. Thus since the sun was God; this meant that God could reach every cell of the body and heal any illness through the celestial body's forces.

In instances of disease or any kind of illness, whether of body, mind or spirit, these ancient people recognized that such did not reside in the physical body but in a higher source. Therefore, the ill were not healed via care of the physical body, but were taken into a higher spiritual place to be healed. There they were placed in a special healing room, which was constructed of a special kind of stone and crystal and was artfully shaped and angled so that the power of the sun was diffused into beams of different-colored cosmic light and energy. Centered in the room, certain sunrays fell on the patients and healing colors were chosen and filtered through the sun and projected onto them under the direction of the priests. The priests of this civilization evolved into a higher state of consciousness and with this power were immediately able to detect the cause of illness and the appropriate means of cure.

ANCIENT SCIENCE AND RELIGION OF HEALING

For a period of time in ancient Egypt, science and religion were closely integrated. Initiates from the priesthood were dedicated to the healing arts. Healers were grouped into three categories: those who were known as the healers of the herbs, and secondly the more scientific healers, such as the surgeons who tended to the afflicted with the knife. Their surgical skills were highly sophisticated, and some of their approaches are similar to what is done today. However, instead of using surgical sutures they used melted wax to heal the wounded skin surrounding the incision. Then the surgical site was wrapped in a cotton dressing that was blessed by the priest. Today, some practitioners of therapeutic touch institute a similar practice by wrapping a patient's wound with cotton cloths charged by the healer's spiritual energy to accelerate healing.

The last group of these healers was psychics who had clairvoyant skills of diagnosis and healing. The high priest of Anubis possessed the ability to see with the eyes of spirit and could look into the body and the auric field as well to diagnose any physical, mental and spiritual abnormalities the afflicted may have been suffering from. Some of these priests were reported to have the power to heal patients with their mind from a faraway distance.

It was written that the priests even had further skills, including the ability to lift the sick from their bodies and place them in an astral projection position prior to surgery. This unique practice eliminated the necessity of pre-surgery anesthesia, which is commonly used in modern medicine. However, the priests did administer certain herbs featuring anesthetic qualities in a drug form.

Overall, the priests were well trained in the healing arts and were innately conscious of the role of the healing spirits. Every kind of illness had its own kind of healing treatment that always incorporated spiritual incantations, thus weaving science and the spiritual healing arts closely together. Actually, the spirits were asked to tend to the healing ritual to ensure successful healing. Thus, side-by-side stood the physician and the priest tending the ill. Existing as one group, scientists and priests follow the doctrines that are based upon the integral scientific knowledge of the human being "existing" as a multidimensional entity. Thus within this philosophical concept the afflicted were treated in the manner which could be equated with today's alternative healing practice.

Much of alternative medicine while appearing as new innovations has heavily leaned upon generations of healing experience. In ancient times, healing occurred in more humble soundings, such as our forefather's kitchens, where strong pungent odors of freshly picked herbs permeated everywhere, while brewing all day in huge metal kettles, or within primitive thatched huts under the shaman's care. While such environments differ, the essence of healing methods is strangely similar to alternative healing. Thus while many view this healing trend as being new and modern, just about all of its techniques existed many years ago. Individual practitioners add their personal approach, but still attempt to maintain the basic roots of the original pattern of care, and incorporate them in their present healing techniques.

Thus, patients have the best of both worlds; that of healing methods that have endured throughout the ages, and those more recently developed various contemporary medical scientists. "New-age" visionaries: Edgar Cayce; Dr. Andrew Weil, Harvard Medical School graduate; Dr. Jay Rowen, medical doctor and researcher from Alaska; Dr. James Whittaker, granddaddy of preventive medicine; and Dr. David Williams, who has traveled all over the planet seeking new cures. Several have written extensively, such as medical textbooks and on various subjects in natural healing. Each is well known in their field, and several have private medical practices. In conclusion, these healers have a great respect for ancient healing, which is integrated within their current practices. To add, Dr. Rowen includes in his care "Color Healing Therapy," a healing practice from ancient Greece, which has proven successful for a number of his patients. (More extensive information on the modalities are covered elsewhere in this book.) Upon request, he will send a rainbow of colors on small acetate sheets and instructs how each color can function for individual ailments. Dr. Weil has several audio tapes on visual healing, a technique derived from the ancient yogis of India, and of course the master of spiritual healing, Edgar Cayce, wrote on ancient Egyptian healing practices.

Each of these healers, borrowing from past ancient healing practices, is closely woven into various contemporary methods used in alternative healing. This encompasses primitive herbal cures, shamanism, and healing methods of ancient civilization, all which have left behind a treasure of healing modalities proving so valuable in alternative healing. Living in a medical technology age, such healing modalities have surprisingly been able to integrate into today's numerous healing methods. For example, some of more common alternative healing practices include acupuncture and massage, which have their origins in China and India, two ancient cultures with a legend of sophisticated healing experiences. In the pioneer days, where professional medical cures were limited, healing remedies basically came from the mouths of women, for some giving connotations as being nothing more than mere "old wives' tales." While unpopular today, older women's leading role in families, such as grandmothers, were revered for their wisdom and also for their knowledge in methods of healing. While younger women were preoccupied with raising children and doing basic household chores, and men were preoccupied with hunting, less active older women were better able to discern cause and effect of any given illnesses and with this wisdom were able to devise the most effective methods of healing.

To add, in cultures experiencing prosperity, where the land was relatively peaceful, where environmental elements were satisfying, and bountiful with natural beauty, usually located near warm bodies of water, such as Hawaii and the Caribbean Islands, matriarchal societies were quite common, with older women often playing leading roles. As healers, older women were revered as earth goddesses or "mother nature." In various Southwest Indian tribes such as the Hopi and Zuni, women were highly revered for their healing, nurturing skills. In the contrast, in violent primitive societies where hunting dictated the lives of the villagers, and perhaps those controlled by certain religious societies, where male "God" figures predominated, gradually, women's voices fell to a whisper, and eventually their healing powers diminished. Left of these past healing remedies, once controlled by women, are healing recipes often passed down within the family. Modern medicine shows disdain for these "kitchen healing remedies," and anything that hints to being "primitive," or "home brewed," or not deriving from orthodox medical science. The reasoning behind this medical scientific attitude is that all healing substances need to go through what is referred to as "double-blinded" testing before being FDA approved. However, these past remedies went through generations of testing and throughout the years have proven their worth.

Another ancient practice integrated into today's alternative healing is what is referred to as "intuitive healing," or what may be called "faith healing," and practiced by the known psychic healer Edgar Cayce. In history, we are told Jesus also used intuitive healing. Actually, Jesus in his many travels carried with him no healing material, and certainly was far removed from any scientific medical or even herbal substances. Only through the use of such resources as what we today refer to as "psychic powers," faith, or "intuitive healing," Jesus was able to look upon a human and determine the illness the individual was suffering from. Interestingly, among primitive societies, as well as American Indians, healing methods used intuitive healing. The healing shamans, highly honored in their society, required many years of devoted training to acquire such skills. Today those in the field of intuitive healing borrow from these ancients, and as in the past, use certain psychic senses to determine an illness. As the ancients and primitives had no tangible means of healing, healers relied on their cognitive skills, and sensitively feeling certain vibration in the patient's voice, along with questioning their mental-emotional state. With this information, healers are believed to be able to diagnose an illness.

EARLY AMERICAN HEALING

Early American settlers brought with them to the new world their precious herbal seeds so that their acquired knowledge and skills would not be lost. The colonists learned from the Native Americans about herbs native to North America, and the cycle continued. An Englishman named Whitaker compiled Native American herbs into an early report sent home with "good news from Virginia." His report included information on the many native plants, including "pines, pitch trees, also cedars, ashes, maples and cypresses and sassafras, which inhabitants referred to as Winauk, and was a kind of wood with pleasant and sweet smell, and rare virtues in physic for the cure of many diseases."

The herbal knowledge of the Native Americans was greatly welcomed by the early colonists, who then knew little about natural methods of healing. Obviously, newly dependent upon local plants for their healing remedies, the inhabitants had a respect for native vegetation. In 1621, an Englishman wrote, "We are told that the Indians are suffering contagious disease, of which Physicians could give no reason or remedy, yet in a short amount of time, was restored to their health merely by drinking water. Saxifrage tea was infused and boiled, which was discovered to them by the natives, and we justly entertain belief that many excellent medicines, either for conservation of Nature, in her vigor, or restoration in her decadence, may be communicated unto us…"

The experts say authoritative research shows that, all told, Native American remedies added fifty-nine drugs to the modern pharmacopoeia. Home treatment of many ills was a way of life during this time in history. Reliance on herbal cures was commonplace.

Unfortunately, some dishonest dealings transpired and not all physicians involved with healing were regarded kindly.

In 1617, the Society of Apothecaries was founded in London. Only members of the society were permitted to keep an apothecary's shop and prepare and sell natural medicines. The society's bible, *The London Pharmacopoeia*, was published in 1618. It contained standardized formulas for the proper preparation of herbal drugs. *The London Pharmacopoeia* was not available to the masses, but the common man benefited greatly from Nicholas Culpepper's *A Complete Herbal*, published in 1649. This work remains a respected report from a master herbalist of the times, and is still widely quoted today.

It must be remembered for centuries that healers of old gathered their own medicinal cures or bought them from locals who either grew and harvested them or foraged local fields. Doctors personally compounded the ingredients from the healing herbs the teas and poultices they dispensed, the formulas of which were carefully guarded. When the apothecary shops first came onto the scene, the physicians wrote prescriptions and the apothecaries filled them, but the doctor still compounded his own medicines. Using a mortar and pestle physicians ground up the medicinal herbs before dispensing them, along with detailed instructions for their use, to their patients.

In 1841, the Pharmaceutical Society of Great Britain was founded and education and training of pharmacists became mandatory. Apothecary shops dispensed standardized herbal compounds, but this was still a dark ages as far as medical practice was concerned. With good reason, the sick feared having to go into hospitals. Most people who went in came out feet first, due primarily to the filth. Unknowing physicians were not conscious of the fact they were carrying deadly bacteria from patient to patient as they made their rounds. Baron Joseph Lister, the famed London surgeon, changed all that in 1865 by demonstrating that antiseptic procedures and basic cleanliness saved lives.

While improvements were made, still "self health care" was the basic healing method used by the people. Herbal medicines and teas were staples in every household. Shops with trained apothecaries were found only in large cities, and published manuscripts giving information on more modern healing techniques were unavailable to the general masses. However, traditional healing herbal mixes and other natural remedies were passed from generation to generation by word of mouth, often referred to today as "old wives' remedies" and thus usually not considered important.

Modern science has long replaced ancient beliefs that most illnesses were uncontrollable, or mysterious aberrations. Home healing remedies and the street peddlers' magical cure-all tonics, popular in the turn of the century, became antiquated during the advent of medical technology.

Traditional medical science, which plays a dominant role in today's healing institutions, adheres to what it regards as the "state-of-the-art" healing, based on the cookbook repetition of previously time-proven methods of drugs and other various medical treatments. Much of the medical practice through the years has been based on what might be known as the scientific medical consensus. What was accepted rarely budged from the safety of the norm. Amid scorn from their peers, lonely medical pioneers would occasionally break this barrier and pull out from that magical bag some innovative healing modalities. However, these healers often found themselves bucking up against the established viewpoint of medical healing.

Ideally the most beneficial means of healing is the integration of past remedies with current medical discoveries thus possibility generating a more comprehensive wave of healing. This would offer more possibilities in curing seemingly incurable medical situations. Thus opening a wider span of healing modalities offers healing possibilities for those who have given up on orthodox medicine, perhaps even having resigned to living with their illnesses. Actually one basic goal of healing of the twenty-first century is representing the integration of the present medical system with a diversity of ancient healing modalities. It would be sad commentary if generations of time-proven healing remedies were pushed aside and forgotten. Nevertheless, we are a nation that throws away the "old," where minimal reverence towards the "tried and true" is appreciated. We prefer to make our own discoveries, always starting from scratch, which can inadvertently throw away valuable experiences. However, as alternative healing expands, remedies that are more ancient will be discovered and recognized as a valuable asset to the growth of medicine of the future.

CHAPTER 8

POLITICS AND NATURAL HEALING

THE BATTLE GOES ON

An active movement has been consistently resisting those practicing alternative medicine, however, true to form, California is taking steps towards protecting the natural health movement, but it is a battle. This most populous state in the country is rapidly moving to restore medical freedom despite the traditional medical board statement, which includes, "physicians will be disciplined for negligence or incompetence" due to any treatment rendered that is considered a deviation from the standard of care. The medical board continued, "The standard of care is determined by the medical community, and the medical board seeks expert opinion to rule if the care was a departure from that standard." The problems for those who ascribe to non-conventional methods is that the standard is set and measured by the conventional medical community, and therefore the care they provide is likely to fall outside that standard. Under present law, the medical board has the responsibility to discipline physicians whose care is outside of the legal level of the standard, even if the treatment was sought elsewhere because the "caused no harm" was ineffective for that particular patient. Without legal protection, those practicing non-conventional methods have good reason to fear disciplinary action. There are those who are looking to prevent this disciplinary action from taking place by supporting the legislation protecting alternative medicine.

For years, a long hard battle has been brewing in keeping supplements from coming under the control of the medical field. For a while, questions were up in the air if vitamins and minerals would be available only with a physician's prescription. Intense protests regarding this resulted in the medical field finally backing out. It truly came as a shock to some that citizens were so openly assertive and so intent on expressing their rights regarding this subject. Politically, the medical field realized the result of lost votes and, knowing where their bread was buttered, dropped the case. However, rumors occasionally leak out that this situation may repeat itself. Those devoted to natural health obviously need to take their stand once again and acclaim their rights to the freedom of acquiring these supplements without the medical establishment's interference.

A Senate bill (S-722) would turn over all natural supplements and vitamins to this bungling bureaucracy. At a time when many citizens are having trouble paying for their medicines, to shoehorn the FDA between them and the "low-cost natural supplements" is considered outrageous. Thus, what is required is that those devoted to natural healing to be continually prepared to protest against such extension of an erring bureaucracy.

Millions of Americans take supplements daily; therefore, is it only natural that there would be complaints made against a particular substance. Some people expect overnight fixes from supplements, because many have resorted to taking them when all else has failed. They ignore the fact that supplements, for best results, need to be taken on a regular basis and some on a long-term basis to prevent the reoccurrence of the illnesses and to completely repair the damages done. Methods used in natural healing heal individuals more gradually than traditional healing, because the former helps to heal the body within. Thus, individuals grow healthier on a more permanent basis because the approach is to flush the core of the particular illness out of the system, rather than temporarily camouflaging it, which is the tendency of most chemical drugs, one of the basic means of healing used by the medical community.

One problem associated with those using supplements is that since they are less harmful or obtrusive than pharmaceutical drugs, overdosing is not harmful. Some users believe that, if one supplement works, then two or three should be better and quicker. Overdosing on anything will cause ill results, whither it is a natural supplement or a chemical drug. However, the repercussions on this is that under the S. 722 bill, only one complaint is required to trigger a call from the FDA to remove all products containing any particular nutrient. A scenario such as this could occur: An individual, stressed out from work, decides to take magnesium to protect his or her heart. After taking it for only two days, he still suffers a heart attack due to long-time stress and poor diet. According to this new bill, the manufacturer must report this incident to the FDA, giving it the authority to take this supplement off every shelf, without any research or testing. This is how anxious the authorities are to rid natural healing supplements from our lives. Now it is up to the manufacturer to prove that the cause of this heart attack had no relation to the supplement, which may take years. The weight loss herb ephedrine is a good example of the time it takes to prove that the supplement or herb is not at fault.

For years, it has been a long hard struggle keeping supplements from the controls of the medical field. For a while, there was question whether vitamins and minerals would only be available with a conventional physician's prescription. Because of a deluge of protests, the medical field had second thoughts. For some medical professionals, it was surprising so many citizens were so openly assertive; intent on keeping their rights continued…they protested. Politically, the medical field realizing they were losing many citizens' confidence, they backed off. However, rumors have been passing around that this situation is not over and it will begin again. Moreover, those devoted to natural health will take their stand, and once more fight to keep their rights.

UNFAIR PROCEDURES

Only one complaint will wipe away a particular supplement. In contrast, a prescription drug would have to cause several deaths and have very serious side effects before the FDA would take any action to remove it. The fact is, prescription drugs kill over 100,000 Americans per year, and maim many times that figure; the FDA pulls very few of these drugs off the market.

Conversely, a minimal amount of people die from supplements, perhaps ten or twenty in the past ten years, and the majority of these deaths result from abuse of ephedra, a stimulant substance which causes severe harm if overdosed. It is in agreement by most everyone that standards that are more rigid need to apply toward supplement companies, to weed out the bad from the good, and to differentiate which health claims are accurate from those that are fraudulent or harmful. This research requires time and money, and most of all the motivation to focus on the many benefits of supplements.

A recent letter written by Senator John McCain read, "The FDA has not done a credible job at regulating prescription drugs. Drugs have been approved that later had to be withdrawn because of adverse effects, even deaths; the costs of the FDA approval process have denied other drugs that might be useful; and the time involved for approval restricts modern medical progress."

We all want to believe the FDA is trustworthy; after all, they are seemingly the protectors of our food and drug industry, but not always do they deserve our complete trust. For example, the FDA requested that folic acid distributors not reveal to their customers that it helped prevent birth defects. However, many refused to listen, and when they became aware of this supplement's benefits, it saved thousands of babies from possible birth defects.

In another case involving the FDA ban of I-tryptophan, a form of vitamin E—in making the vitamin, it was believed that a batch somehow became contaminated, causing harm to some of its users. Even though later it proved the culprit did not originate from the supplement, the FDA stuck to their guns and placed a skull and crossbones on everyone who even mentioned the case. Consequently, we still do not have access to this wonderful healing supplement. In the meantime, a study recently published, reported that hundreds of deaths occurred from the use of a major drug used for healing the flu. No move was made to take this deadly drug off the market because, first it would require months, if not years, going through legal litigations and accusations against the reverential and powerful drug company producing it. In the meantime, after the ban of I- tryptophan, the alternative physician Jonathan Wright continued to prescribe it, and because of his defiance, the FDA raided his office. When he filed suit, the FDA retaliated by storming into his clinic with armed sheriffs, who terrorized employees and ransacked his medical supplies and records, seizing as much as they could, and almost drove Dr. Wright out of the medical business. Realizing the unfairness of this attack, the doctor filed suit in district court, charging unlawful search and seizure and demanding his property. In response, the FDA convened a federal grand jury and subpoenaed his clinic records; no charges were ever filed.

Another case chronicles the famous raid on the Bursynski Research clinic in Texas on July 7, 1985. Due to this doctor's alternative and noninvasive treatment of cancer, NCI, Aetna insurance, and others who had pressured the FDA into throwing their weight around instigated this unjust raid. They indiscriminately seized over 20,000 medical and research records, forcing Bursynski to make copies of them, at his own expense, while the government tore through his building searching for evidence they could use to make their accusations stick. Again, the FDA filed no charges in court.

When the government, for a second time, made attempts to ban the free marketing of supplements, 24 million angry Americans signed petitions, the health stores, libraries and most other public places provided a place to congregate; with concerted effort people inundated Congress with letters, faxes, and telephone calls. The FDA knew it had no alternative but to back away from this proposed ban. However, this showdown created the Dietary Supplement Health and Education Act, which specifies the powers the FDA has over the nutritional supplement industry.

The actions of the FDA often appear less to do with the health and safety of the public and more with politics. With additional power, they would then be in control over every supplement manufactured. Approval would have to come from the FDA; then, obtaining vitamins legally would only happen through a prescription from a medical doctor. Not only would this be costly, it would consume copious amounts of time, because it would require patients to make appointments with doctors, keep the appointment and then travel to the local pharmacy to purchase the supplement. It would be at the doctor's discretion in making the choice between writing a drug or supplement prescription, and from past history, the former is the preferred choice. Such a system would remove individuals from making their own choices, thus minimizing their role in being responsible for their own health.

PROTECTING YOUR RIGHTS

Some believe that sometime in the near future the freedom we now enjoy in using nutritional supplements will be in serious jeopardy. Under the dubious guise of "consumer protection," the S. 722 bill before the Senate could give bureaucrats complete and unchecked control over the supplement industry. A while ago, a movement began to curtail access to the wonderful curing herb echinacea, which everyone in natural healing regards as a healing gem. Like any substance, if used incorrectly, echinacea can perhaps produce negative effects. The basic problem is if used too extensively, echinacea loses its effectiveness. This herb's miraculous healing quality is its ability in helping to resist colds, flu, sinus and other infections, thus minimizing the use of antibiotics.

Meanwhile, the movement to ban echinacea was nearly successful, and to this day, some still stick to their guns, emphatically refusing it, regardless of proof of its effectiveness and thus, prefer using harsh drugs. The question is why use harsh drugs when gentle healing herbs will do? It's like "killing a mosquito with a shotgun," particularly when a beautiful flowering plant grown from God's earth can do the trick safer and with less damage to the body. What makes matters worse is doctors prescribe antibiotics for almost every ailment, which not only have negative side effects but also lose their effectiveness after a period of time. This can be a "catch 22," meaning that if a life-threatening infection occurred, the body and the disease can become immune to antibiotics. The bottom line is that doctors should prescribe powerful antibiotics for emergency infections and illnesses only and not for minor flus and colds. Listing the numerous side effects of pharmaceutical drugs, such as damaged livers, kidneys, destruction of the body's own immune system and many others, so often hidden from the public, outweighs any problems supplements may have. For example, in order to read the side effects a popular over- the-counter drug for flus and colds, hidden underneath a label on the bottle lists many…some pretty serious. In the meantime, customers unaware of these dangers possibly would not have purchased it. Certainly, no one is going to rip off a label on the medicine bottle before purchasing, which no doubt, the manufacturer is relying on. Such greed and deception is unforgivable.

Few people realize that drug companies fork out millions of dollars to the FDA to obtain approval for their drugs; that doesn't include the wining and dining.

There is a possibility supplement companies may find themselves doing the same thing in order to have FDA approval and to keep their products available to the public. Such control will devastate those committed to natural means of maintaining their health, even to the point of getting rid of their doctors. For some, after unsuccessfully seeking relief from a stable of doctors, finally arrived at the point of relying on themselves and the supplements and herbal cures they take. Thus for those dead set against returning to the orthodox healing world, the availability of these supplements is absolutely crucial and should at all times be available to them. In a free democracy, any tampering with an individual's method of choosing to heal themself is unconstitutional; take legal action.

CHAPTER 9

ALTERNATIVE HEALING AND CANCER

Cancer research and treatment has become a booming industry. It has been said that more people make their living off cancer research than those who die of it. Billions of dollars have been poured into what some believe to be a bottomless sinkhole in the search for a cancer cure. While some cancer researchers have become rich and even famous, those seeking means of alternative approaches towards cancer prevention go unrecognized. Yet nothing close has come to solving the cancer dilemma. Even the Congressional Record has acknowledged little progress has been made. Conventional therapy has proven to be a dismal failure, as the rapid spread of cancer keeps growing. A documented case of "complete cancer cure" through chemotherapy is nonexistent, and yet it is the most dominant therapy offered to cancer patients in this country. In the meantime, some discoveries both in the use of less invasive therapies than chemotherapy, and cancer prevention have yet to be introduced to the mainstream of cancer cures for the simple reason the medical establishments denies their validity. One reason is that focus is directed towards attempting to heal patients after they become sick, rather than approaching preventive cancer methods.

It is common knowledge while the medical field produced an assortment of so-called "heroes" in their claims of coming close to a cancer cure, lacking is a successful conclusion. To add, pharmaceutical drug companies' strong ties to cancer research programs have stifled the budding of some unique findings rationalizing they were not FDA approved. Hence, the politics of cancer therapy has been as bad as the disease itself, causing much conflict and a wide separation between conventional cancer treatments from those practiced by alternative healing practitioners. Often it was the work not of medical doctors but individuals in other healing fields who made pertinent discoveries in cancer prevention, while bucking the system.

Even today, with the evidence that some types of cancer can be prevented through the executing of a certain lifestyle, many cancer specialists vehemently deny such findings. Comprehending and accepting such simplistic concepts regarding cancer prevention such as the adherence to a strict nutritional regime, along with selected supplements and herbs, including practicing certain healing modalities and avoidance of emotional stress, is difficult for those relying only on medical science for cures. Even further, vehemently denouncing their validity, the medical establishment went as far as accusing those promulgating such notions as being dangerous to the public and effectively had rounded up a few alternative-healing practitioners and put them out of business. That left just three "accepted" therapeutic approaches to cancer: surgery, chemotherapy, and radiation, "cut, poison and burn."

Those in alternative medicine, realizing the difficulties involved in completely ridding the body of cancer once it has entered the system, promote the necessity in taking preventive measures in avoiding it. In the meantime, cancer treatments are approached with more gentle remedies, which are virtually nontoxic, and at times more effective than conventional chemotherapy. No doubt natural means of approaching cancer treatment requires thoughtful and creative approaches, and above all time and patience. This is because a large diversity of treatments is formulated to suit the individual needs of each patient's chemistry, type of cancer and its severity, and also the level of the patient's inner strength. To add, for those having weak physical systems, heavy doses of chemotherapy can counteract the healing process and weaken patients even more. Actually, there are studies which prove cancer can be slowed down without the use of harsh approaches, by simply minimizing the use of chemotherapy. The key here is to strengthen cancer patients' systems by building up their immune system so as to prevent the growth of cancer cells and to keep them from spreading.

At the Aidan Clinic in Tempe, Arizona, under the auspices of Dr. Daniel Rubin, patients are anxious to tell their success stories. It appears that the program initiated by Dr. Hugh Riordan and his father, Neil Riordan, who worked with hundreds of people during the 1900s, included a study on the effect of vitamin C on cancer. What they discovered was that vitamin C enhanced the activity of the immune cells. Administration of intermittent high doses of vitamin C induced remission in such cancers as kidneys, lymphoma, and small cell lung cancer. By 1995, vitamin C emerged as an effective therapeutic agent. Alternative health individuals made the breakthrough in the discovery that cancer cells are vulnerable to vitamin C, which is perhaps the most common vitamin that most of us take on a daily basis. Such innovative research rids of the concept that cancer can only be cured by chemotherapy.

HEALING VISIONARIES

At a recent medical conference, Dr. Steven Ayre of Chicago gave a presentation on a more novel way to administer chemotherapy, which was nontoxic and more effective. Many years ago, this doctor became aware of the work of a visionary Mexican physician who was using the hormone insulin, even before the age of antibiotics, to treat and cure a myriad of diseases, from syphilis to cancer. Traveling back and forth to Mexico, Dr. Ayre observed, and was instructed on, the technique by the physician descendant of the pioneer, Donato Perez Garcia, MD. The next step was to try to understand how the administration of insulin prior to exposing cancer to chemotherapy would make the cells so much more sensitive, so that only a fraction of the conventional dose would be necessary to get the desired effect. The positive result of Insulin Potentiation Therapy was because chemotherapy doses were so small that normal cells were left unharmed. Normally, chemotherapy harms healthy cells along with the sick cells in the body.

So compelling was Dr. Garcia that the Mexican Secretary of Health recommended further study of IPT. The Mexican army established an experimental clinic to do just that. Dr. Garcia then made a trip to Tijuana in the San Diego area in 1944 and treated many diseases, including syphilis, malaria and even a gallbladder disease. *Time Magazine*, on April 10, 1944, documented this trip in a short article. When penicillin was widely used in World War II, the same year as the development of IPT, this type of treatment became obsolete as treatment for syphilis. However, Dr. Garcia continued to work with IPT as a treatment for other diseases.

In 1983, Dr. Garcia III, at the family practice, joined Dr. Garcia II. In 1987, both doctors treated their first AIDS patient with IPT and an antiviral drug. The patient reported a reversal of symptoms and returned to health. IPT treatment is not available to patients in the United States, but there are now nine doctors actively using IPT therapy throughout this hemisphere. The big discovery for the IPT treatment was with cancer patients. It was found that it helped make cell membranes more permeable to other substances including chemotherapy drugs, enabling more drugs and insulin to enter the cells. Strangely, even with these discoveries, there are very few facilities in the United States that use this type of treatment. However, they are used throughout Canada and Europe, where there are no restrictions by the US FDA on alternative healing treatments.

Dr. Robert J. Rowan, a medical doctor from Alaska and alternative health practitioner, gives one case history of an elderly male with lung cancer that used this treatment. When this patient had suffered two other cancers, it was recommended he receive full doses of chemotherapy, but instead, he chose IPT treatments. As proven by CAT scans, cancer was growing each month prior to IPT; after IPT started, there was no longer any growth of a tumor. Thus, treatment was reduced, and after two months of treatment, there was no evidence of further tumor growth. Developing some temporary hair loss and a slight fall in blood count were about the only sacrifices this man made for the exchange of regaining his health and becoming cancer free.

THE HEALING OF A PROMINENT DOCTOR

Dr. William R. Fair sought out alternative treatment for cancer he suffered during the period when he was a hotshot head of urology surgery at a famed cancer center in New York City. Dr. Fair, who not only was trained under the conventional medical field, and was also head of a cancer center that utilized traditional treatment for cancer, including foremost the use of chemotherapy, contacted another alternative doctor, Dean Ornish, MD, who is nationally known for his statements that "dietary and lifestyle changes alone could reverse heart disease," and who saved Dr. Fair's life.

When Dr. Fair discovered that he had cancer, his longtime suspicions of its existence were confirmed. Being a doctor he understood the symptoms but was in self-denial and ignored what he knew was in inevitable. The cancer was surgically removed but it had already spread. This particularly nasty type of cancer that Dr. Fair was suffering from was bad enough; following the surgery and a year of chemotherapy, the tumor reappeared. It was then a decision was made to attack this cancer and go in a different direction. Dr. Fair worked with the group of researchers in attempts to develop a special vaccine based on his specific cancer cells. However, the most productive move was following a healing regime suggested by his friend, Dr. Dean Ornish, a well-known alternative medical doctor. Dr. Ornish was able to convince a very prominent conventional cancer physician of the urgent need to change his former type of treatment. Urging the doctor to attend the Cancer Help Program at Bolinas, California, along with a week-long retreat to learn coping strategies, spiritual direction, yoga, and meditation, Dr. Ornish insisted that his friend find some time each day to meditate. This very traditionally trained doctor initially looked upon these suggestions as being just a little bit "kooky"; after all, Dr. Fair was the head doctor in a highly established cancer center that followed very stringent cancer treatments, which excluded any form of alternative healing, so with great reluctance, and some skepticism, he finally attended the retreat.

Dr. Fair also contacted Sophie Chan, PhD, a researcher and associate professor at the Brander Cancer Research Institute at New York Medical

College. Dr. Chan had been working for years with a Chinese herbal combination called SPES (Latin for "hop") that was showing great promise against cancer. As it turned out, Dr. Fair knew about this treatment and thus decided to try it. Since he had been taking SPES, scans showed progressive shrinkage of this cancer. In the meantime, his personal experimental vaccine is still on the shelf.

It is obvious that this doctor made a great transformation through alternative medicine, which he had one time questioned. He also credits his healing to a personal metamorphosis into the realm of spiritual beliefs and his general attitude towards life. He has learned to rid himself of his former workaholic attitude and to retain inner peace acquired from daily meditation sessions. In summary it was through the adherence of a stringent course of healing approaches responsible for Dr. Fair's cure, which included dietary changes, a lower-fat diet with lots of fruit, vegetables, and whole grains, and as well as stress relief, meditation, Chinese herbs, and all contributing factors. He then commented in humor, "I now seem like those California hippies I used to make fun of, but I really had to experience it myself." Like so many other people, Dr. Fair turned to complementary medicine out of frustration with conventional medicine.

During this time, Dr. Fair claimed his doctors were relentless in getting him to continue with conventional chemotherapy, even though it was not working for him. Soon after, Dr. Fair left Memorial Sloan-Kettering after sixteen years to join his son in developing a national chain of complementary health facilities, and act as associate editor of the journal *Alternative Therapies and Health and Medicine.*

NO MORE BREAST BIOPSIES

A young woman painfully winced as her breast was placed on a plate, squeezed and flattened out like a pancake as she was preparing to receive a "low-intensity" X-ray called a mammography. She claimed it felt like her breast tissues were being torn apart. Later she told her doctor she would never get another mammogram, despite a strong family history of breast cancer. Mary is one of millions of women encouraged by the breast cancer scare to subject themselves to the rather brutish mammogram tests. This procedure includes the mechanical flattening of the breasts in order to acquire the best picture, since imaging through thick tissue can often obscure the result.

At the time, Mary was unaware of the availability of another screening method that is highly accurate, which does not use radiation and is far superior at preventing breast cancer than are mammograms, which never prevent...just diagnose the disease. Digital Infrared Thermography works like this: the average body temperature is 98.6 degrees, which is measurable due to the metabolic and blood vessels' activity in the body. This is why thermography is so successful. This type of test observes function (metabolic activity) by heat observation and detection whereas mammography uses penetrating X-rays to observe structure.

Thermography has been around for decades, but few doctors prescribe it to their patients even though it is much more advanced breast testing technology than standard mammography. In 1982, the FDA approved thermography as an adjunctive diagnostic screening procedure for breast cancer. Since then there have been thousands of screens done and a multitude of reported studies, the results of which are startling. The average sensitivity and accuracy in detection of the disease of breast thermography is ninety percent. In comparison, mammography carries a sensitivity rate below eighty percent and often as low as sixty-five percent. Thermography can also give a risk assessment of future development of breast cancer far more accurately than family history because you can see the metabolism shift in action. It can be used to assess success of early intervention before cancer develops. Dr. William Amalu in California, who has an active screening clinic, claims this advanced technique can detect any disturbances in the breast area up to ten years before cancer actually develops, thereby enabling women extended time to take preventive measures if needed.

Preventive measures are much more effective because breast tumors in early stages can be treated, whereas once cancer sets in it is much more difficult to treat. In addition, thermography protects women in the age bracket of thirty to forty years who tend to get yearly breast exams from cumulative effects of radiation from mammograms.

Finding a doctor who practices this procedure may prove difficult since they are rare. However, a local imaging center should be able to help locate someone who practices thermography. Whoever does the imaging should be board-certified, and not limited to just being trained by the company that sells the device. Another source to contact is the International Academy of Clinical Thermology, which lists qualifications of technicians and interpreters, and also provides a list of qualified centers worldwide. Since thermography is just a test measure, and not a cure-all for cancer, it has its limitations.

FIGHTING BREAST CANCER

Another testimony concerns a young woman named Nancy Brinker who, learning she had breast cancer, decided to fight this disease and do whatever it took to overcome it. Creating a foundation for breast cancer called the Susan G. Komen Breast Cancer Foundation located in Dallas, she went to work battling this disease. Raising more than $2 million, this foundation became the world's largest private foundation of breast cancer research. Ironically, one of the first lives saved by the foundation was Nancy's own. Nancy insisted that her doctor no longer do any more biopsies and refused to have the tumor removed from her breast, but her doctor was reluctant because he felt her life was at stake. He became even more anxious when Nancy described to him what her plans were for healing.

Starting on an intensive natural healing program, Nancy followed her own self-healing practice. It included prayer, and doing a lot of visualization, which involved filling herself with bright white light and visualizing her cancer cells melting away and with this, she added a daily dose of laughter, which she discovered was so beneficial. Her intensive yearly checkup showed that, more than fifteen years later, Nancy was still cancer free. Still following her natural health regimen, which includes taking plenty of vitamins and using herbs to help boost her immune system, walking four to five miles each day, following a Mediterranean- style diet, and incorporating some humor in her life, she feels she is well on her way to preventing any future problems.

A few years ago, many people felt the idea of alternative medicine was taking a multivitamin and maybe some vitamin C and of course garlic. However, people like Edmund Rubin, a seventy-six-year-old retired department store buyer and manager, are alternative medicine personified. When, in 1990, he discovered his kidney cancer had spread, he decided to take extreme action in use of natural remedies. Despite experimental treatment with interferon, a second aggressive tumor appeared above his left ear; the tumor was treated unsuccessfully with radiation. His weight dropped from 135 to 105 pounds. The doctors did not tell him what the medical reports said, "he had just six months to live." Rubin knew he had to do something.

NICHOLAS GONZALEZ, MD

Rubin heard about Nicholas Gonzalez, MD, a New York City physician who was said to be successfully treating incurable cancer with an intensive program called "The Gonzalez Regimen." By this time, Rubin was so wiped out that he was willing to try anything, even going as far as experimenting with this "crazy stuff." By then his regular doctors had given up on him, so he started the program. In six months, Rubin's weight went back up and his tumor disappeared. The exact level of effectiveness of this treatment was undetermined since some patients expecting overnight miracles dropped it when failing to reach their expectations. In addition, other patients when feeling better after a few treatments believed they no longer needed further treatments, but then their cancer returned. As for Rubin, the inconvenience and difficulties of continuing with it were worth it. Determined to get well, he stuck to the regimen.

This included taking 150 pills a day: vitamins and minerals, granulars and extracts, and huge doses of specially designed pancreatic enzymes; he is "cleansed" daily by several coffee enemas. The former steak and spaghetti lover—"You couldn't get me near broccoli," he admits now— eats a nearly vegetarian diet and consumes a quart of fresh carrot juice every day and almost everything he eats is organically grown. Rubin admits all this is a lot of work and requires a lifetime commitment, but quickly adds it is worth it because it saved his life.

THE GONZALES REGIMEN

This special cancer program was devised from Dr. Gonzalez's treasure hunts through forgotten conventional medical literature. As a second-year medical student, he came across the work of John Beard, MD, a Scottish embryologist and biology professor at the University of Edinburgh who, in the early 1900s, observed that the placenta, the organ that supplies nutrition to the growing fetus in mammals, looks like cancer at the cellular level; unlike cancer cells, placenta cells stop growing on cue. That cue was the pancreatic enzymes secreted by a fetus, Dr. Beard discovered. Obtaining these enzymes from slaughterhouses, he injected them into animals with cancer and reported that the tumors just "popped off." Dr. Beard, using enzymes to treat cancer in humans, achieved cures, as documented in medical journals in 1911.

After Beard's death, Dr. Gonzalez and a couple of other doctors, all considered crazy by the medical establishment, attempted to carry on his work, which resulted in a great success, and word spread about Dr. Gonzalez's cancer work. In 1993, the National Cancer Institute asked him to present a test case of patients' recovery of cancer. In the pilot studies, Dr. Gonzalez chose eleven cancer patients expected to live only three to four months, and upon completion of his treatment, all but two lived for at least two years and two lived more than four years. Among them was a woman whose breast cancer had spread to her brain and liver and after undergoing this treatment her cancer went into remission. Impressed, the National Center for Complementary and Alternative Medicine at the National Institutes of Health awarded Columbia Presbyterian Medical Center in New York City a $1.4 million grant to adopt a study comparing Dr. Gonzalez's regimen to chemotherapy on cancer patients who suffered a grim prognosis. The trial recruited people in New York City and seven enrolled and took the Gonzalez Regimen for some six months; all but one is still alive. A clinical nurse, M. J. Gaybay, who recruited patients for the trial, claimed several of them were doing quite well though she cautioned that too early conclusions may prove inaccurate.

Such highly unorthodox cancer treatments brought an onslaught of harsh criticism, which included a sharply negative story on Dr. Gonzalez and his protocol, which was published in the *Washington Post*. Only time will tell whether the Gonzalez Regimen is the answer for curing deadly pancreatic cancer and other forms of this disease; perhaps with more proven tests and positive results, the answer will be revealed. (Those interested in learning more about cancer and ways to beat it, or about Dr. Gonzalez and his therapy, can call number 212-213-3337. To join the pancreatic cancer clinical trial currently underway at Columbia Presbyterian Medical Center the number to call is 212-305-9468.)

DIET, EXERCISE, NUTRITION, AND CANCER

Basic means of cancer prevention, agreed upon by alternative practitioners, is adhering to a strict diet and this is the fundamental way to start. Researchers at Johns Hopkins University reported that three-day- old broccoli sprouts, which are tender shoots, are loaded with the concentrated form of certain powerful cancer fighters. The study showed that there is up to fifty times more anti-cancer chemical in broccoli sprouts than in the mature vegetable, and the sprouts really don't taste like broccoli, which is fortunate for the palates of most.

"Actually, your diet can cause cancer," warns Dr. Andrew Weil, a great advocate on maintaining good health through eating right. Even though you may think your diet is good, it may have certain damaging substances probably overlooked. First, barbecued and smoked meats have been proven to cause cancer, as well as some drinking waters. Dr. Weil claims the ideal diet, particularly if fighting a serious illness, is the macrobiotic diet, a simple diet, made up of unprocessed brown rice, steamed seaweed and green leafy vegetables, as well as beans, grains, and tofu. This diet excludes meats, sweets, starches, and fruits. Some find such a diet unappealing, particularly those who enjoy rich spicy foods; however, like any food one has to acquire a taste for it. Dr. Weil also adds that the right kind of oil is extremely important to include in

the diet to prevent cancer. Recent research at the University of Toronto has shown that flaxseed oil reduces cancer of the breast and also colon cancer in rats. A Spanish research team recently set out to discover whether olive oil, fish oil, and safflower oil would prevent cancer. Their findings suggested that olive oil and fish oil might help protect against cancer, but that safflower oil failed the test. As for cancer and diet, Dr. Weil claimed the basic problem with most diets is the large amount of refined carbohydrates and sugars consumed. These foods are not easily digested, and in many cases become glue-like in the digestive tract. To see how this works, Dr. Weil suggests mixing a little water with some refined flower, which is the main ingredient in breads and pasta, until you get a nice paste. Put the paste between two pieces of paper, and when dry, attempt to pull them apart. It will not be long before the two pieces of paper are inseparable. (This glue is perfect for craft making since it has such a strong bond.)

SUPPLEMENTS AND CANCER

Dr. Andrew Weil agrees, with other nutritional experts, that another cancer fighter is supplements; several nutrients he says are necessary include magnesium, CoQ10, garlic, zinc, vitamin C, selenium and folic acid. He adds that, when you are suffering from a particular ailment, other supplements can be taken; a good nutritionist would be able to advise you on the best supplement to take. A research study involving 1,312 patients was conducted over a period of six months, half of whom received selenium and the other half receiving a placebo. The selenium-treated group had sixty-three percent fewer cases of prostate cancer, fifty-eight percent fewer breast cancers, and forty-five percent fewer lung cancers. This result concluded that selenium resulted in an enormous decrease in cancer.

Another cancer fighter, which is rarely brought up because of all the cancer hyperbole connected with it, is sunlight. Contrary to those who promote the idea that sunrays are unhealthy, sunlight is a healer. Obviously, certain precautionary measures need to be taken, such as the use of a good sun block and limiting the time of exposure. However, sunlight is a powerful healer for many afflictions, including the emotional ones, and provides an excellent source of vitamin D, which is necessary for proper calcium absorption. Americans are inundated with caffeine substances, from coffee to soft drinks, which are most people's first choice of drink. What is so shocking is that, although a multitude of data proves caffeine causes cancer and also hypertension, our schools and children's recreational facilities still feature soft drink machines, offering an array of caffeine- loaded drinks. Although parents have been battling the problem of ridding their children's environments of these soft drink canteens, California and New York are the only two states that have legally removed them from schools' property. Some question the fact that feeding our children these caffeinated beverages at such a young age may be setting them up for future ailments and complications. To make matters worse, the average school cafeteria is loaded with fried foods, starch, and sweets, which officials claim is needed to make foods appealing so kids will buy. This money is needed to keep up special programs; so in essence, we are slaughtering the lambs for the sake of money.

Pediatricians report that children at an earlier age than ever before in history are suffering from illness caused by poor eating habits, especially diabetes, cholesterol problems and even cancer. Actually, these diseases are becoming an epidemic with children in United States. The question is for some, how we can expect the continual smooth running of a nation if our future generation is constantly ill.

EXERCISE AND CANCER

Another cancer fighter is so simple many doubt its effectiveness—that is exercise. While most know the general health benefits of exercise, many still avoid it. A recent study found that walking at a normal or brisk pace for one hour per day is associated with a forty-six percent reduction in risk of cancer. With the variety of exercises that have emerged, even the most sedentary can join in with some type of exercise. Along with walking, swimming, running, and gym work such as lifting weights, various forms of stretching are vital, but often overlooked. Health specialists claim that yoga, known as an excellent means of stretching the body, is beneficial in keeping the body strong, thus keeping the immune system working better, an essential factor in warding off cancer.

Recently another form of exercise, called Qigong, has surfaced, which has proven to be beneficial for health maintenance. In China, there are healing centers referred to as "medicine-less hospitals" which use Qigong along with Tai-Chi, acupuncture, and herbal cures for curing diseases as severe as cancer. Dr. Tom Wu, a medical physician from San Francisco, works along with Master Paul Dong, a Qigong practitioner; Qigong has proven this particular energy practice is practically beneficial in helping cancer patients.

Of Chinese origin, Qigong is best described as a powerful healing art, which empowers individuals to gather Qi from the environment and circulate it within the body. This is done through breathing mechanics, magnetic field strengthening, meditation, and moving energy along specific meridians. Since the energy feelings of Qi can be so strong, practitioners use it in their healing treatments of all kinds, including cancer, for the simple reason that supplying the body with more energy helps to combat illnesses.

The primary theme of Qigong practice is internal energy "storage," something we all can use. Actually the practice of Qigong enhances strength by this "storing of energy" where it then can be directed and then activate when needed, particularly when the body is struggling with a physical problem. It awakens special abilities from the surplus vital energy in the brain and in a way, can be responsible for individuals to live up to their full potentials because they have the physical and mental energy to do so.

Qigong is the backbone of the entire Oriental culture and the seed for all martial arts systems, acupuncture, Feng Shui and Chinese medicine. It was traditionally recommended for children, beginning at the age of seven, within royal families. Besides royalty, the 6,000-year-old art form was rarely shared outside of special family bloodlines. However, recently the secret exploded and now in mainland China, there are about 300 million Chinese practitioners.

No doubt, alternative medicine and treatment offers hope for some major diseases considered terminal or incurable at one time. Now they are viewed as being treatable, sustainable at a reasonable level, and curable. Aside from cancer, diabetes, high cholesterol, high blood pressure, acute cases of crippling arthritis, those prone to chronic infections, and poorly functioning immune systems, have a chance for recovery and without undergoing harsh medical processes. As an increasing amount of alternative healing clinics open their doors, and include focusing on cancer healing, further research into cancer with the use of alternative healing methods can emerge. Rather than considered as the last resort, which is so often the situation with cancer patients, alternative healing can become the first choice of seeking a cure.

In conclusion, alternative healing is responsible for manifesting a more positive approach towards such grave diseases as cancer. Differing from the past where the mere mentioning of cancer immediately brought up images of "incurable and deadly," a more productive attitude is being taken. Alternative healing enables cancer patients to have a better grasp on their illnesses, and nurtures a sense of hope of recovery as they become aware of the various healing methods available to them. As more possibilities open up in cancer research in the field of alternative medicine, patients can expect to be treated with less invasive methods that are "more human friendly" than orthodox treatments. After all, is that not what cancer patients really want and need in their hour of despair? However, the acceptance of the medical establishment is needed for alternative medicine to be able to make any significant headway in cancer cures that will be readily acceptable by the public. It is only hoped this will occur before too many more lives are lost to this disease.

CHAPTER 10

THE POWERFUL PHARMACEUTICAL COMPANIES

The street was packed
With desperate believers, so in need of relief, Of their lifetime illnesses
And, the man selling snake oil made a killing...

TOO MANY DRUGS

(U.S. prescriptions have swelled by two-thirds over the past decade to 3.5 billion yearly.)

Many individuals are inundated with pharmaceutical drugs, prescribed by their own physicians. Most lack the slightest inclination of what they contain, and their side effects, some can be quite deadly. Yet consuming them like candy, millions of Americans are oblivious to their dangers. Recently the news media came out with a report on several of these life- threatening drugs and gave descriptions on individual deaths that resulted from them. In the meantime, while there was an initial scare, it appears Americans are not listening to these warnings and the consumption of pharmaceutical drugs still remains high. Many people become drug dependent and suffer from drug addiction because they take several medications at one time. A health worker in a nursing home reported that patients would line up in front of her station an hour before her arrival, going in hysterics if she was one minute late, demanding their medicines as if they would drop dead if deprived of them.

It is quite common for physicians to be drawn in when a prestigious research study on a particular drug has been finalized, toting with fanfare of its potential for miraculous healing, particularly if it promises to cure some serious illnesses, such as cancer. Doctors are pushed on by persistent and convincing pharmaceutical sales representatives, hovering over their doorsteps with loads of free medical samples, with the intention that the doctor will generously offer them to their patients, who will eagerly accept the free handout. Of course, when these freebies run out, they will automatically be prescribed to patients, who then have to foot the bill, while drug companies' pockets get fatter.

Thus doctors get caught up with the pharmaceuticals because their years of study in their medical careers have programmed them to believe more in the medicine and less in the healing, which has made some so arrogant that they feel no need to write out legible or legal prescriptions; the free stuff will do the job. Now we all know doctors can write legibly, or how in the world were their college tests and terms papers written.... Okay, computer word processors can be used as an excuse for their poor handwriting, but the older doctors, the ones that have their own practice, did not have computer word processors while going to medical school.

At the very moment patients complain about their health problem, regardless of how minor, expectations are they will leave their doctor's office with one or more prescriptions in hand. Actually, patients have come to expect getting these prescriptions and even may feel cheated if they are denied. Doctors realize this, thus they attempt to give patients what they want. A prescription can somewhat appease a frustrated patient, particularly if the doctor has been unable to exactly diagnose their problem. This attitude inevitably perpetrated the recent crackdown pertaining to various medicines prescribed to patients that make claims of their benefits of healing a whole range of diseases, which there is proof they could not. Fortunately, this residue of "snake oil" was scrutinized and banned. Drugs companies are inhibited in making claims of curing ailments beyond the scope of what they were originally intended.

Pharmaceutical drugs, for doctors, are a predominant part of their healing methods, thus a new promising drug on the market can almost be mesmerizing; it does not help that drug companies wine and dine doctors. A recent incident included a newly drug, hot on the market, was being over-prescribed to patients from their doctors. The question was why this drug was being prescribed for so many different ailments, particularly for those that over-the-counter remedies could be just as beneficial. Actually, doctors rarely prescribe over-the-counter remedies, concluding that they are inferior to prescription drugs. Of course, this is not always the case. Usually, it is best to support a healing remedy that is the least invasive to patients, which obviously would start by giving advice on good health habits, diet, exercise, taking certain supplements; then go further by prescribing the mildest remedy possible.

For the simple lack of supervision, there are many situations where patients overdose on drugs. For example, when patients are unable to acquire a particular drug from their doctor, they just seek out another doctor that will fill their prescription. Most physicians do not take the time to check if their patients are loading up on a particular medicine. This loading up can be particularly dangerous if the prescription they seek is a "controlled" drug. In addition, aging patients can forget their schedule of taking their medicine and thus, unnecessarily repeat taking it.

WORKOUT

Listed below are precautions to take when taking prescription drugs.

1—Avoid taking prescription drugs unless it is an extreme illness, and you have no other choice.

2—When a particular drug is prescribed, its side effects need to be researched, such as asking the pharmacist and searching the Internet. Also a book called *Consumer's Guide on Prescription Drugs*, by Peggy Boucher Mullen, Pharmaceutical Doctor, offers comprehensive coverage and gives information on hundreds of brand-name medications and their generic equivalents, as well as how to talk to your doctor and pharmacist about them, how to administer the drugs, and coping with their side effects.

3—Inquire from an alternative health professional what supplements you can substitute for a particular drug that may have been prescribed to you.

A medical physician that practices alternative healing would be ideal. They will recognize, when taking a stronger drug, it is essential for them to check if there is a gentler cure that is more appropriate; the latter is usually preferred.

4—Research less invasive cures that are better than drugs, such as approaching a good herbal naturopath physician or Oriental healing herbalist, who often combine acupuncture treatments or homeopathic healing with the use of certain other healing remedies.

When taking a pharmaceutical drug, always search for the least strong dose, and try to take the least amount in the shortest period of time. Try not to get hooked on taking any medicine for a long period of time; you want your body's own defense mechanism to work. If you do not see results with a drug within six weeks, or the side effects are too overpowering, it is the wrong drug.

TESTIMONY

Alice and Ken Heckman each begin their morning by cracking open a rattling plastic tray carting scores of pills in a rainbow of pastel hues. Between the two of them, they gulp down twenty-nine pills every day; a regimen of fourteen drugs, with a chaser of dietary supplements. With all this, the Heckmans are fairly healthy, but believe without their reliance on their drugs, their lives may come close to a halt; they are that addicted to their drugs. Curiously, about 130 million Americans, many far healthier then the Heckmans, swallow, inject, inhale, infuse, spray, and pat on prescribed medication daily, as the U.S. Centers for Disease Control and Prevention indicates. Americans buy more drugs than any other nation.

The pharmaceutical industry served up more than $250 billion worth of sales last year, the vast majority in prescriptions, according to industry consultants. That roughly equaled sales of all the country's gasoline stations put together or an $850 pharmaceutical fill-up for every American.

The question lies, do we need all these drugs? While a handful of drugs may be lifesavers for certain conditions, many common ailments are unnecessarily being treated with them. Due to highly intensified promotion of drugs, just about every ailment, such as daily life conditions, aches and pains, antacids, allergies, depression, shyness, premenstrual crankiness, waning sexual powers, impulsiveness in children, you name it, it is a candidate for a drug prescription from doctors. However, virtually all these common ailments have potentials of being successfully treated with changes in diet, exercise and other natural means.

"We are taking way too many drugs for dubious or exaggerated ailments," says Dr. Angell, former editor of the prestigious *New England Journal of Medicine* and the author of *The Truth About the Drug Companies*. "What the drug companies are doing now is promoting drugs for long- term use to essentially healthy people. Why? Because it's the biggest market."

To add, relatively few pharmaceutical newcomers greatly improve the health of patients over older drugs or advance the march of medicine. Last year, the Food and Drug Administration classified about three-quarters of newly approved drugs as similar to existing ones. Thus, drug makers churn out and promote drugs with the same ingredients in a different form for a different disease. What makes these drugs sell so well is that patients, unable to get results from the present drugs they are taking, assume a new drug "hopefully" will give better results. Individuals suffering from ailments are more vulnerable, thus, more likely to grasp onto anything that promises a cure.

HOW SAFE ARE THESE DRUGS?

Recently numerous reports have come out on the safety of various drugs used for treating depression, and anti-inflammatory drugs, pushing Vioxx and Bextra from the market. Statin drugs for lowering cholesterol were reported to have caused deaths, yet not a month later, another pharmaceutical report came out toting the benefits of statins in the possible prevention of colon cancer. In the meantime, more than 125,000 Americans die from drug reactions and errors each year, according to Associated Press projections from *Landmark Medical Studies*. That could indicate pharmaceutical drugs as being the fourth-leading national cause of death after heart disease, cancer and stroke.

Drug safety researcher Dr. James Kaye of Boston University said he remembers a medical schoolteacher telling the class: "All drugs are poisonous."

Ken Heckman found out on his own how true this statement was when he lost his alertness for several months to a depression medication and his wife came down with a rash from one heart medicine and muscle aches from a statin drug. Hospital patients suffer seven hard-to-foresee adverse drug reactions and another three outright drug mistakes for every 100 admissions, estimates Dr. David Bates, a researcher at Boston's Brigham and Women's hospital. That translates into 3.6 million drug misadventures per year.

CASE HISTORY—A SAD STORY

Doris Morris, a retired schoolteacher, is taking seven different FDA-approved prescription drugs. The side effects of each drug caused another problem for which her doctor had to prescribe another drug, and then those two drugs caused more side effects, and another drug was prescribed to treat these ailments and the scenario carried on until she was taking seven drugs daily. Now you would think this teacher would be smart enough to realize what she was doing to herself, but just like so many other individuals, she had been brainwashed to believe and follow exactly what her doctor prescribed. Doris started to suffer from a serious case of gastroiditus, which her doctor was unable to cure, which in all probability was the result of all the drugs she was taking. In her blind faith, following her doctor's instructions, she saved enough money from her teacher's retirement fund, which is limited, to say the least, to take a trip to Mayo Clinic. Those who have any experience with the Mayo Clinic know very well that they are devoutly connected to the conventional medical field and emphatically deny any notion of alternative medicine. In a way, this is almost criminal, for the simple fact that many severely ill patients resort to the Mayo Clinic after they have searched the planet for medical help. Too often, these desperate patients have not received the benefits they could have if alternative means of healing were considered by this prestigious clinic.

There is no doubt pharmaceutical companies have taken advantage of their leading role in medicine, which is no doubt the result of the high costs of medicine. A book written in 1984, titled *The Medical Industrial Complex*, by Stanley Wohl, MD, of Stanford Medical School, stated Dr. Wohl's observation of the rising power of the pharmaceutical industry. Lela Lilyquist, one-time certified surgical technologist, claims, as an employee in a county hospital, she saw greed firsthand. For example, she said she had questioned the surgeons and the role of the pharmaceutical companies that were funding a study of abdominal surgery in which a patented pharmaceutical substance (that was substantially just common bleach) was used to irrigate the abdominal cavity prior to sewing up the surgical incision.

How did our surgeon justify going along with this ploy? How could such a blatant act of physical destruction occur right in front of a surgeon? Was it denied that bleach, while it may kill germs, could also kill or seriously damage a patient?

HARMFUL DRUGS

Again there is additional news on the deadly effects of FDA-approved drugs. After many years since Prozac, Zoloft, Paxil, and others have been on the market, antidepressants finally are being labeled, "take with caution," after several teenagers who were prescribed antidepressants committed suicide; obviously this warning came too late for those taking such drugs. The vote to put the strongest possible warning label on antidepressant prescriptions marks a turning point in the heated debate about *all* drugs. This all came into effect after enough anxious parents accused the government's lack of taking strong enough measures in informing the public of certain possible side effects of pharmaceutical drugs, the most extreme being suicide. While parents emphatically claim their children's suicide resulted from the antidepressants they were using, still doctors denied this to be so. Their defense is that their patients suffering from depression would be worse off if these drugs were unavailable to them. This sounds like a repeated theme where parents criticize doctors over-prescribing antibiotics and Ritalin to their children, which again such drugs resulted in harmful side effects.

Obviously, the quickest method of medical care is prescribing antidepressants to depression patients. To help patients, doctors formulate certain beneficial programs, making counseling and psychiatric treatment available for potential suicidal victims. Included in such programs would be closer observation on how these individuals spend their time. The programs recommend that teachers communication more with parents, who may have potentially troubled children and teens; teaching them good health habits and engagement in group stimulating activities and projects that students would be responsible for to lift their self-esteem. The teachers and doctors would monitor these levels of entertainment programs, checking to see if their patients and students are physically well and getting enough sleep and exercise. Last, but not least, domestic issues, which may be responsible for child and teen depression, need to be taken into account. In other words, such patients should be treated holistically, mind, body and spirit, instead of quickly pushing those suffering depression onto medication. In conclusion, a thorough evaluation of patients' unique problems and devising a particular program suitable for them all, which takes time, is essential.

A BIG MISTAKE

Pharmaceutical companies are responsible for the great errors they made regarding a cure for menopause, a natural change in women's lives, when they convinced women that menopause was a disease, an affliction due to estrogen deficiency. Then they fired off a campaign that women could regain their youth and health by taking excessive amounts of estrogen and synthetic progesterone, to be taken by all women from menopause to death. What a powerful market for their talented and able core of advertisers! To add, they managed to do this over thirty years, making billions of dollars per year without ever having to prove that the treatment (called hormone replacement therapy, HRT) was beneficial or safe.

An article written in *New Times Naturally* warned about the harmful effects of synthetic hormonal therapy and the growing awareness of more natural approaches. It seemed the traditional medical field was still taking the lead and not listening to this "safety" message regarding the excess harm caused by HRT. Suddenly, left with no alternative, the Women's Health Initiative Study of HRT using Prem-Pro was halted mid-stride due to the excessive harm from the use of this drug combination. The question now stands is why was this harmful combination permitted to be given to women over thirty years without the drug companies having to prove its safety? Are they so powerful they were able to convince the Food and Drug Administration?

DRUG FUNDING OF MEDICAL SCHOOLS

This is but one example of the power now wielded by the pharmaceutical companies. One physician stated that when he was in medical school at the University of Minnesota in the early 1950s, the medical school funding came mostly from three sources: student tuition fees provided about thirty percent, another thirty percent came from profit in treating patients at the medical school clinics and the hospital, and thirty-five percent came as a subsidy from state coffers. That has changed drastically; the recent *Minnesota Medical School Bulletin* revealed that the state now provides less than eight percent of the school funding, the largest funding for the medical school deriving from pharmaceutical companies in the form of grants for research…desired by the drug firms.

A report made by Carol L. Roberts, MD, president-elect of the American Holistic Medical Association in Brandon, includes how the pharmaceutical companies have a strangling stronghold on medical students in virtually every medical school in this country. Our major universities' medical schools have been, in part, supported by drug companies and rely on their research funding where individual companies will research a particular drug they are touting on the premises of the particular medical school in which medical students take part in the research. Medical students and doctors are continually brought up-to- date on the latest data for new drugs. Being inundated with this type of information and environment, it is no wonder family physicians become hooked on drugs for their patients and often write prescriptions for very young children, convincing their parents that their children's survival depends upon a particular prescription medicine.

Unfortunately, many parents in the lower income bracket, uneducated in any self-help health maintenance, rely solely on their doctors for their children's health care. Too often, rather than offering general commonsense good health advice in means of preventing illnesses, children are immediately put on prescriptions with minimal advice on health prevention for the simple reason doctors believe that such information is not only irrelevant but that uneducated parents will be unable to follow such advice.

One example is the situation with Ritalin been over-prescribed for children with attention deficit disorders, rather than seeking other means to calm children, like getting them away from the television, listening to destructive music, playing destructive videos, watching their diets, omitting sugar; they can increase the consumption of fruits and vegetables while practicing emotional healing and talking to the child with patience and love. Teaching meditation, introducing certain hands-on hobbies which the child can focus on for a length of time, and changing children's environments, making them more calming, all will help to eliminate attention deficit and stress. These emotional problems are not natural byproducts of the human system, they stem from the surrounding conditions in which we place the individual. Thus, rather than prescribing a narcotic drug to children, the root cause of this problem needs to be scrutinized before an appropriate lifestyle formula can be prescribed for the individual.

CONTROL OF DRUG COMPANIES

To add, research findings that do not favor the drug firms usually remain unpublished. Thus, having valuable medical research get in the hands of powerful pharmaceutical companies that are in the position to censor whatever they want, curtails the "freedom of information" and uses the information for profit; this conduct would not be permitted in other disciplines. More important, medical education, where teaching is controlled by pharmaceutical hierarchies, also places huge limitations on how and what the medical students think, thus leading them to treat their patients with unnecessary amounts of drugs. Since drug companies are huge financial sponsors of these institutions, complying with such deceptive situations insures further financing, and denying the pharmaceutical companies would actuate the demise of any medical establishment.

Pharmaceutical companies control doctors' education throughout their medical school years, and thereafter, influence the way they approach their practice. It is mandatory that physicians attend at least fifty hours of accredited continuing medical education (CME) every three years. Now agreeably, this is a good thing, since medical science is always coming out with new research, but there is a catch to this scenario. CME only counts for accredited seminars, in which the accrediting process is controlled by the American Medical Association. An interesting question comes up regarding who at the AMA decides which seminars to accredit. There exists a panel of people inside the AMA, with controlling power to pharmaceutical companies, that makes the accrediting decision, thus, CME-accredited seminars are bombarded by pharmaceutical propaganda for new drugs.

Adding this control in the medical schools' seminars, the heavy-handed drug companies, in the publication of medical journals, along with frequent visits and gifts to the doctors, plus loads of free samples of drugs, which doctors shower onto their patients, convinces the doctors of the quality of their product, thus increasing the number of prescriptions, and company profits. Your health pays for the name of this game. This is a very profitable process for pharmaceutical companies and they have no intentions of stopping it.

MORE CONCERNS

Suddenly, three drugs that proved to be very effective treatments for arthritis started causing anxiety in their users. Many of these individuals went from confirmed believers to skeptics, anxious about their very lives. The FDA-approved medication that was killing people. This current wave of concern reveals the truth in how drugs are handled. Over-hyped commercials flashing on TV screens, with promises of particular drugs offering complete cures, render drugs, either over-the-counter or pharmaceutical drugs, as a mere commercial commodity. Thus, it is shocking that something so vital as medicine is exploited by commercialism. As long as drug companies inflate the value of their dugs through the media, the public will be denied clear objective information about the drugs they are taking.

Regarding Celebrex and Vioxx, the public was ramped up by direct-to- consumer advertising (a selling method permitted only in New Zealand and United States.) This form of advertising is not adequately supervised by the Food and Drug Administration, and the public was misinformed that the so-called "Cox Inhibitors" protect the stomach in a way other non-steroidal drugs cannot, all of which can cause bleeding ulcers and gastritis in their users. Celebrex was considered a potential wonder drug, and hundreds of thousands of sufferers were taking it; that is, until the recent news of its deadly side effects aired all over America.

Even when individuals are aware of the many different alternative healing methods, they still head straight to the pharmacy with a handful of prescriptions. Most doctors scoff at any means of alternative healing... actually some get very defensive and warn their patients to stay out of such dangerous nonsense.

DIRTY DRUG MONEY

Recently, the news media reported a pharmaceutical scandal on how a particular drug, Neurontin, was touted by Pfizer to be a "cure all." Neurontin is commonly prescribed for migraine headaches, attention deficit disorder, restless leg syndrome and even bipolar disorder. It appears, patients have been victimized by Pfizer's unethical efforts to persuade doctors to prescribe the epilepsy drug for "off label" use.

It is not easy nowadays to claim the trophy for "Most Despicable Corporation Activity," given the competition, but Pfizer is a leading contender. The world's largest pharmaceutical company, Pfizer pleaded guilty to misleading doctors and patients on the number of diseases that could be treated effectively with its epilepsy drug Neurontin. While Pfizer has agreed to pay $430 million fine, that is a trivial amount compared to this company's ill-gotten profits on this drug. Pfizer points out that the illegal promotion occurred before the company acquired Warner- Lampert, the maker of the drug. While this may be so, Neurontin remains one of the most in-demand drugs, with annual sales of $2.7 billion, and the bulk of that is for what is called "off label" use for ailments other than epilepsy, which it was intended for; this was the only use for which the Food and Drug Administration approved the drug. This drug is still being prescribed for migraine headaches, attention deficit disorder, restless leg syndrome, and even bipolar disorders, for which it is no more effective than a placebo. Pfizer issued no warning in its news release about the settlement or the ineffectiveness of this drug.

What is so harmful is the fact doctors participated in this swindle. By law, drug companies are not permitted to promote off-label drug use, but are allowed to suggest drugs for the use of variable conditions, but only under very tight scientific evidence that it will prove beneficial for such an illness. However, that has not been the case with Pfizer; many doctors accept benefits from this drug company, which includes paid trips to conferences.

To make matters worse, some doctors were allowing drug representatives to accompany patients in the examining room to promote their drugs to them. According to the *New York Times*, drug companies continued to hire ad agencies to do clinical trials, and then pay experts to put their names on ghostwritten studies and hire physicians as consultants to influence other doctors in the drug choice. In the past year, at least seven drug companies have been investigated for promoting off-label drug use and it seems to have developed into an ongoing problem.

Since the FDA backed off from this aggressive enforcement of the law, this deceptive practice has free license to continue at free will. However, with the court's victory over Pfizer, this attitude may change. The basic motivation is the cost the government has been carrying, such as Medicaid payments for off-label use of Neurontin, which runs into millions of dollars. Where these patients could get inexpensive over-the-counter drugs for many of these ailments, Medicaid has been paying for a more expensive drug, which patients did not need. In other words, "where an aspirin would do," Neurontin was prescribed.

DRUGS SALES PITCH

A 2002 study in the *New England Journal of Medicine* showed that direct-to-consumer advertising amounts to sixteen percent or more of all spending on drug promotion. In 1997, the FDA issued a series of feeble guidelines and permitted TV ads with only a brief mention of negative side effects of any given drug. Since then pharmaceutical companies have had free rein to create the most outrageous TV and magazine ads, campaigns, they most always belt out gross misinformation. The FDA receives approximately 32,000 requests yearly from drug companies for approval of television ads, which makes it impossible to weed out those unworthy for public viewing. What makes matters even more horrific is that some drug TV ads have gone so far as to promote unhealthy lifestyles such as the consumption of fatty foods and sugar for those suffering from cholesterol and sugar diabetes problems because individuals had available to them a drug that would cure these diseases.

The bombardment of prime-time TV commercials proclaiming the merits of particular drugs that cure any illnesses, viewed in clinical-like surroundings to promulgate their validity, brings in millions of "wanting patients" to the doctor's office, increasing pharmaceutical profits by billions. To go further, viewers are encouraged to continue with their present unhealthy lifestyles because these advertised drugs will cure whatever ails them. One particular commercial even promotes irresponsible eating habits to individuals with cholesterol problems because the drug they are toting promises to cure them. Of course, there is no mention made pertaining to following a healthy diet to prevent cholesterol occurring in the first place. Obviously, this irresponsible attitude on the part of a media, which holds enormous powerful influence over its viewers, is based on viewer rating greed. The media gives not a thought to motivate their viewers to follow positive health practices.

AGGRESSIVE MARKETING OF DRUGS

Not a week went by since the FDA was found negligent in permitting deadly drugs to go on the market, when another new drug was promptly announced to the public, as being both effective and safe. This miracle drug, Lunesta, used for insomnia, reported to be safe even when used for a long period of time, promotes its benefits of giving a full night's sleep. In mid-December, the Food and Drug Administration approved this prescription and the drug's manufacturer is planning a $60 million campaign to take the news directly to the sleepless in advertisements wedged between reruns, classic movies, and political gabfests. Companies will buy a lot of advertisement, and this drug is expected to be one of this year's most heavily marketed medications. The public is again caught on the bandwagon of TV drug commercials, and the promises of yet another miraculous drug that makes promises to be safe. The question you should ask yourself is "If this drug fulfils its promises and is as miraculous as it promulgates, then shouldn't word of mouth suffice?" The drug company is taking no chances and wants to get as many customers as they can purchasing this drug and perhaps getting hooked on it, although they claim it is not habit forming, which is to be questioned since even natural sleep remedies are habit forming. This new sleeping aid in medical parlance is called eszopiclone. It is a hypnotic drug which, in itself, indicated addiction. While many eyes will be focused on Lunesta, some skepticism is in order.

The news regarding the harmful effects of various popular drugs, particularly the arthritis painkillers Vioxx and Celebrex, both approved by the FDA, has left many wondering of this giant's validity. After all, if you can't trust the FDA to keep our food and drugs safe, who can you trust? Perhaps this is just another indication of the growing number of institutions becoming incapable of serving the public. However, when lives depend upon this agency's abilities to do things right, it's imperative they can be thoroughly trusted in doing just that; too often, the public receives nothing from the FDA but shortcomings.

TESTIMONY

Dr. Marc Siegel, an internist and associate professor of medicine at New York University School of Medicine, writes in the *St. Petersburg Times* of his experience with a representative from Pfizer, the drug manufacturer of the most of these harmful drugs. He claims that the very day that Vioxx was removed from the market a Pfizer representative was stationed in his office hallway attempting to convert him to prescribing Celebrex instead to his patients. Outraged, and being an outspoken New Yorker, Dr. Siegel exclaimed, "Have you no shame? Don't you know these drugs have similar effects?" The representative argued that Celebrex didn't have the same problem as Vioxx. A few weeks later, Pfizer pulled its advertising on Celebrex. (No more TV commercials of Olympic figure skater and old household name Peggy Fleming, who epitomizes health and endurance, and her claims on the wonders of Celebrex.) However, the FDA didn't see it fit to withdraw this drug from the market, even after a study showed it raised the risk of heart disease. Then a few days later, concerns were raised of the safety of yet another drug, Naproxen, best known as the over-the-counter Aleve.

What makes matter worse is that it is getting more difficult to make the right choice, and to know what to believe. To add to this dilemma, the federal government's efforts to police the drug ads have not been able to keep up with the influx of the growth of drug advertising. Drug companies spend about $1 billion a year, nearly a third more than they did five years ago, to market prescription drugs to the general audience, publications, and even more to advertise on television.

Ads that show allergy-free people running through grassy fields and satisfied women after their husbands "saw the doctor" about sexual dysfunction, are intended to fuel the demand for brand-name drugs. While commercials are good at designing super-alluring promises of cures, they tend to leave out information on the side effects. The Food and Drug Administration, whose responsibility it is to ensure such ads are truthful, are just plain careless and reluctantly to get overly strict with wealthy and powerful drug companies. This carelessness enables some drugs to slip by without notice, until they harm or kill several people.

Although few people are knowledgeable enough to weigh the risks and benefits of prescription drugs, much less understand the combination of them, the FDA's standards of clarity for print ads date from the 1960s. Back then, drug ads appeared almost exclusively in medical journals and were intended only for physicians. As a result, the so-called "brief summary" to warn consumers of the possible health risks of drugs can run as much as 2,000 words and be as difficult to understand as your doctor is when they prescribe the drug to you. For example, they include such unintelligible sentences as, "HMG-coA reductase inhibitors interfere with cholesterol synthesis and theoretically might blunt adrenal and/or gonadal steroid production." No doubt, print ads for prescription drugs need to be more readily intelligible to the average consumer. However, drug companies have minimal incentive to respond to FDA complaints, because the agency is not taking the responsibility and power it has to seize undesirable drugs and take the money and time to go through court procedures.

The FDA's most common sanctions for a problem ad is a "notice of violation" letter, which directs drug companies to curtail their way of advertising. For serious problems, or repeated offenses or violations which may prove harmful for the public's health, a letter is written threatening to take the drug off the market; this rarely occurs and is becoming even rarer. However, on the other end, a harmless supplement which may face a consumer's complaint will be immediately taken off the market and there will be no investigation.

This is not to indicate there are not times when drugs have their place; today's advanced science has resulted in procuring some very sophisticated medicine, some considered life saving. However, in an advanced diverse society, there needs to be more healing options than the present narrow perspective of pharmaceutical drugs. This is where alternative medicine plays a vital role. The ideal way to approach whether to take a drug or not can best be determined by a physician who practices both orthodox medicine and natural healing. Under such an expansive approach, patients are being treated by a medical doctor who can determine if natural remedies will be effective and if not, then resort to pharmaceutical drugs. This healing method may prove to be the best healing method, and should be initiated into every doctor's training regime. In the future, it may be that most of our doctors will be trained in natural healing, along with having a background in orthodox medicine. Hence, this will enable them to treat their patients with a broader range of medicines, thus alleviating the overuse of potentially harmful pharmaceutical drugs.

CHAPTER 11

HANDS-ON HEALING

NOTHING IS AS HEALING AS A HUG

Over the past hundred years, the healing ministry of the church has gradually diminished. In Europe, healing was once referred to as the "royal touch." Kings from several countries were reported to have healing power that they used on those suffering such diseases as tuberculosis by the method of laying on of hands. For several centuries, this method prevailed, starting with Edward the Confessor and ending with the reign of William IV. Jesus predicated belief on the healing powers of kings who had certain rights and privileges endowed to them.

In 1778, a radical healer daringly pronounced that he and he alone without faith in spiritual healing was able to heal. His name was Franz Anton Mesmer, and his theory was based on what he termed an enlightened use of universal energy called *fluidum*. He came to believe that all physical bodies, animals, plants and even stones, were impregnated with this magical fluid that gave them special powers and was responsible for their healing. He reported that the life-sustaining and regulating actions of the magnetic fluidum were integral to the basic processes of health. When an individual was in a good, balanced state of health, he or she was considered to be in harmony with these most basic laws of nature. However, if disharmony occurred between the physical body and these forces, illness resulted.

Mesmer came to realize that the best source of this universal force was through the human body and that the palms of the hands themselves contained the highest energy power. For example, the practitioner placed his or her hands on the patient's own, allowing healing energy to flow from one to the other. Some healers even use their fingertips to connect with patients' fingertips and, feeling the heart pulse, connect to this healing energy. While this is a subtle healing enactment, the results can be powerful. Due to Mesmer's influence during the revolutionary period in French history, the technique called the "laying on of hands," otherwise referred to as "magnetic passes," grew popular. Unfortunately, at the time, there was controversy that Mesmer was merely using an act of hypnosis to obtain positive patient feedback.

Healing with the use of laying on of hands has many biblical connotations. Of course, Jesus comes to mind when considering the relevancy of such a healing practice. Few think of questioning his healing of the blind man, the dying child, and many of those suffering diseases in his time when medicine was so limited. We all know how it was simply the power of his touch that healed. Yet, these same believers have a difficult time swallowing the idea that healing can be accomplished by the energetic magnetism that runs between one person and another. It appears that in some ways medicine is stuck in the medieval era in terms of beliefs regarding healing. The medical field cannot accept anything as intangible as touch healing because it cannot be seen or measured. The sophistication involved in the concept that all bodies contain natural healing properties that connect to the universe sounds too unreal for some, yet too often, there has been evidence of healing through just such an esoteric practice.

The use of laying-on-of-hands techniques to heal human sickness dates back thousands of years in human history. In ancient Egypt, evidence of its use can be seen in the Ebers Papyrus dated about 1551 B.C., which describes laying on of hands for medical treatment. The Greeks also used therapeutic touch in their Asklepian temples for healing their sick. The ancient writings of Aristophanes give details of this method of healing to restore a blind man's sight and to return fertility to a barren woman.

Many references are reported in the Bible of healing by touch for both spiritual uplifting and physical healing. Actually, laying on of hands was as common a practice as preaching the gospels, and practicing parts of the sacrament. Combined with the use of holy water and oil some believed that the washing of Jesus' feet, while symbolizing a humble act, also served a practical purpose of hands-on healing such as tending to His ailing feet, with washing and rubbing with the oil after a strenuous day of walking and preaching. In those times, this method of healing was essential since there was little medicine available. This ancient hands-on- healing approach was believed then, as is today, that the cuddled baby is a healthy baby. While in breast-feeding, babies are healthier not only because the mother's milk is believed to be superior to the regular milk formula, it is also the fact that breast-fed babies are held when being fed.

Denied the many medical techniques of today's healing, natural means of healing were utilized; ancient people depended upon what was immediately available to them. What derived from the earth, such as plants, comprised the bulk of the ancients' medicinal remedies, and various hands-on techniques such as massage, cuddling, or bending and twisting a patient in various positions to release the demons responsible for the illness, and was the healing tools used by the medicine man, whose hands contained healing powers. Whatever he touched was magically transformed into a state of good health. With just a tap on the head from the shaman, a patient could expect to be endowed with the blessings of health.

Obviously, much faith and belief in the shaman's abilities to emit such healing powers had to be unconditional. One had to believe in order for the shaman's touch to be effective and since everyone was aware of his long dedicated preparations in perfecting his healing craft, the shaman was totally trusted. The shaman was deeply immersed into the spiritual life, which was ingrained in any method used in healing his patients. Thus, he was honored for his healing powers because he was adored as a spiritual leader. Whatever the shaman touched had to have healing magic. As a holy individual, his very body was the embodiment of this power.

This attitude is evident in various modern hands-on healing techniques. Those in the practice of such healing modalities like massage therapy, Reiki, reflexology, prayer, hands-on healing, and even acupuncture often integrate spiritualism into their healing techniques to obtain the best results. Hands-on healers are aware of the importance of touch as a means of healing, and recognize that some individuals suffer certain ailments as the result of lack of touch. Studies have shown that crack-cocaine babies, that is, those born while their mothers were engaged in doing drugs, were able to become more emotionally stabilized and physically stronger merely by the handling and coddling of them. In war-torn countries where many children were left as orphans, and thus experienced lack of any form of touch, there was not only an increase in diseases affecting immune systems, but also trends of such children tending to be non-responsive, and even expressive of various emotional and mental afflictions.

TOUCHING AND THE IMMUNE SYSTEM

Studies show that touch elevates the immune system, helps alleviate depression and just gives an overall feeling of well-being. However, many are unable to find such comfort within their immediate environment. We are a society "on the go," and little time is given to such considerations. In the past more mothers being home when kids came home could welcome their children with a hug; now today parents are rarely themselves home at such time. Where mothers at one time lovingly breast-fed their babies, which consistently produces babies with higher I.Q.s and healthier immune systems than bottle babies, many mothers are opting for the convenience of formula. In addition, breast-fed babies grow up endowed with stronger bonding abilities and are generally more emotionally stabilized. To add, busy mothers now often leave their babies with childcare individuals, who may hurriedly thrust a bottle of milk into the baby's mouth without the slightest care. We are not a hugging society; we are filled with busy schedules, with little time for what sadly, may be considered incidentals; touch is vital to our well-being and should be considered a major health factor in our lives. That is one of the reasons why various hands-on healing techniques have become so much of a healing trend.

POINTS TO CONSIDER

1—Make certain you feel comfortable with your healer. If you don't feel completely relaxed, the benefits will be minimal. You need freely communicate your problems so the healer can determine the correct approach to take. However, some hands-on healers do incorporate prayer into their healing, and thus at those times it is best to remain silent, perhaps with a low-volume chanting or meditative music playing in the background.

2—Make certain, as you should with all healing environments, that everything appears to be sanitized. Many illnesses spread right within the doctor's examining room and healing areas. Some who practice alternative healing may be less focused on hygiene basically because their training background does focus on clinically sanitized conditions.

3—You need to find out if the hands-on healer employs a Christian orthodox spiritual healing or other spiritual means and if they are compatible with your beliefs. A more generalized spiritual approach is usually taken, devoid of focusing on any particular religious sect. If you are seeking Christian spiritual healing, you can approach various local churches to see if they offer such information. The Christian Science church is a good place to start. Just beware what you are doing. For example, if you are seeking a Christian approach you may be offended if your healer starts to chant prayers to Buddha.

4—Reiki hands-on healing is an excellent approach, although Reiki practitioners differ extremely. Some use direct hands-on healing, such as Reiki, acupressure and touch, while others use more meditative prayer, which can complement other alternative healing methods.

Researcher Maxwell Cade in England discovered the existence of a biorhythm entrainment between healers and patients. He used a special device known as the Mind Mirror, which is a computerized EEG (electroencephalogram) power spectra analyzer. Cade was able to detect a unique complex brainwave pattern occurring between the patient and healer. However, this only occurred with advanced healers. These unique healings that induced brainwave synchrony patterns between patients and healers were measured both when the two were close together and were separated at a distance. What is even more miraculous is that more involved in the distance praying; the more effective the outcome.

Hands-on healers usually incorporate some type of spiritual prayer or utterance while attending to the patient. In the healing room, an aura of spiritualism permeates throughout, where the patient usually becomes captivated or lost; this is part of the deep relaxation for which the practitioner strives. Through certain music, attractive visual surroundings and a sense of deep quietness, the healer places the patient at ease. The practitioner needs not only emit a sense of confidence but also be able to express compassion and concern for the healing session to be successful. If patients feel uneasy for any reason, no matter how excellent the treatment, the effectiveness is minimized. Unlike orthodox healing, patients' emotions play a vital role in the healing process. Any stress, inhibitions or doubts block the passage of healing from the healer to the patient.

It is pertinent to remember that illnesses can originate at many levels of our multidimensional anatomy and not just at the level of the physical body as traditional doctors view illness and thus treat their patients accordingly. No doubt, there are many surface diseases that attack us, bacteria, viruses, environmental toxins and carcinogens, which, it's important to note, are less likely to attack when individuals are not only in good physical condition but mentally as well, which is rarely recognized by doctors.

At the spiritual level of human consciousness exists a level of perfection and energetic balance with which we all have been endowed and which cannot be affected by distortions of mind and emotion. It is the fundamental law of life and nature that individuals should experience a balance of well-being for a certain period of time on this planet. However, many never experience this, due to unnecessary afflictions often caused by one's self due to ignorance or blatant neglect. While the outer physical body of a person may be experiencing illness, the inner being and inner Idea is quite healthy and seeking to heal the substance, pattern, and function of these bodies. Thus, the ability to heal is an innate human potential. The higher self is always attempting to connect with the physical level so as to maintain good health. Following this reasoning, it becomes obvious that the mind regulates physical well-being. Additionally, it is the spiritual mind that dominates over all.

The ability to heal is an expression of a deep inner desire by the individual to help or heal another through compassionate concern. This empowers the healer to perform successfully various healing modalities, without the use of doctors or medicine. The experience of connectedness between the healer and patient, through unconditional love as Jesus showed in his healings, is a level which must be reached and addressed in the healing professions for greater healing to occur. More health-care professionals need to learn how to activate their inner healing potentials so as to shift healing into a better-balanced and gentler system. Alternative healing offers some approaches that can begin to connect the irrational schism between the material and spiritual dimensions of human existence. However, in a growing materialistic world, we still have a long way to go.

CHAPTER 12

ACUPUNCTURE

Because of the increase of the use of acupuncture for various ailments, practiced not just by Oriental practitioners, but Western healers as well, a complete chapter has been devoted to this subject. To begin, this healing practice is one of the oldest, most commonly used healing procedures in the world. Originating in China more than 2,000 years ago, acupuncture did not become known in the United States until 1971, although it was commonly practiced throughout Europe years earlier. When *New York Times* reporter James Reston wrote about doctors in China using needles to ease his abdominal pain after surgery, some amazed readers began searching for practitioners in the United States that could use this method to heal their ailments.

Acupuncture has grown rapidly in popularity in the United States in the past two decades. A Harvard University study published in 1998 estimated that Americans made more than five million visits per year to acupuncture practitioners. The report from a Consensus Development Conference on Acupuncture held at the National Institutes of Health (NIH) in 1997 stated that acupuncture is being widely practiced by thousands of physicians, dentists, Oriental acupuncture physicians and other practitioners, for the relief or prevention of pain and to alleviate a wide diversity health conditions. Actually, acupuncture is used not just for physical ailments but for mental problems as well, such as depression, since it supposedly raises the brain's endorphins. The NIH has funded a variety of research projects on acupuncture. The National Center of

Complementary and Alternative Medicine (NCCAM), the Office of Alternative Medicine (OAM, NCCAM's predecessor) and other NIH institutes and centers awarded grants for study in the field.

Traditional Chinese medicine theorizes that there are more than 2,000 acupuncture points on the human body, and that they connect with twelve main and eight secondary pathways called meridians. Chinese medicine practitioners believe these meridians conduct energy, or *Qi* (pronounced as "chee"), throughout the body. Qi is believed to regulate spiritual, emotional and mental and physical balance and to be influenced by the opposing forces of yin and yang. According to traditional Chinese medicine, when yin and yang are balanced, they work together with the natural flow of Qi to help the body achieve and maintain health. Acupuncture is believed to balance yin and yang, keeping the normal flow of energy unblocked, and maintain and restore health to the body and mind. Since many practitioners imbue their practice with spiritualism, this attitude is also imparted with the acupuncture treatment. Topics covered by acupuncture treatments include diet, herbs, massage, and meditative mental and physical exercise, all of which are intended to improve the flow of Qi.

There is a difference of opinion of the subject of Qi, and some are not convinced it exists at all. Western scientists have found meridians difficult to identify because meridians do not directly correspond to nerve and blood circulation pathways. However, acupuncturists believe that meridians are located throughout the body's connective tissues, which is a theory followed by the discipline ever since ancient times. Obviously, such controversy was hushed up a bit when the FDA began approving acupuncture treatment for various ailments, particularly the ridding of pain. Acceptance of this kind of treatment reached its peak when insurance companies, who just previously scoffed at any form alternative healing, started to pay for acupuncture.

EXACTLY HOW IT WORKS

There have been various explanations on how acupuncture works. Basically, acupuncture points are believed to stimulate the central nervous system (the brain and spinal cord) to release chemicals into muscles, the spinal cord and the brain. These chemicals either change the experience of pain or release other chemicals, such as hormones, that have an influence on the body's self-regulating systems. This biochemical change may stimulate the body's natural healing abilities and promote physical and emotional well-being. There is still much unknown about acupuncture because, since it is still regarded as a new age and experimental medical practice, studies of it have not kept up with the pace of traditional medical studies. If there were a hint that acupuncture could cure cancer, more interest in the value of this procedure would emerge. However, keeping the bodily system well balanced and maintenance of self-regulating bodily functions so they are in good shape, as acupuncture does an excellent job of, is taking the right steps in cancer prevention.

Probing needles into the human body at certain unseen meridian points still appears too mysterious for some for it to be taken seriously as a means of healing. There are three main mechanisms of acupuncture:

1. Conduction of electromagnetic signals. Evidence shows through studies that acupuncture points are strategic conductors of electromagnetic signals. When these points are stimulated along these pathways through acupuncture, electromagnetic signals are relayed at a greater rate than under normal conditions. Such signals may energize the flow of pain-killing biochemicals such as endorphins to certain sites where the body is more vulnerable to ailments.

2. Activation of opioid systems: Research has found several types of opioids may be released into the central nervous system during acupuncture treatment, thereby reducing pain.

3. Changes in brain chemistry, sensation and involuntary body functions. Studies have proven acupuncture may alter brain chemistry by changing the release of neurotransmitters and neurohormones. Acupuncture has been documented to affect the parts of the central nervous system related to sensation and involuntary body functions, such as immune reactions and processes whereby a person's blood pressure, blood flow

and body temperature are regulated. Pre-clinical studies have documented acupuncture's effects, but since they seem not to coordinate with Western medicine standards, they tend not to be regarded as decisive conclusions.

According to the NIH's Consensus Statement on Acupuncture, it is widely practiced in the United States as a therapeutic intervention. While many studies have proven its usefulness and many valid conclusions have derived from the practice of this ancient Eastern healing method, the mere fact that it did not develop under Western medical standards has always put it to question. Western medicine is reluctant to give the stamp of approval to any form of medicine not committed to black-and-white proof, that is, what can be proven by their stringent standards. Thus, the subtleness and mysteriousness of Eastern medicine is approached with suspicion and derision. The issue is further complicated by the growth of sham acupuncture groups who promise overnight fixes. Acupuncture can be a slow healing procedure since it works with the body to heal itself. Often it requires months of treatments, which alone can be a deterrent for some who are urgently seeking relief, particularly from pain.

While the traditional medical field still views acupuncture with ambivalence, in China it is considered state-of-the-art in healing. Acupuncture walk-in clinics are everywhere, and are used as frequently as are the many fast-noodles cuisine shops for a noon lunch. For a few dollars, a patient can get a quick treatment by a full-fledged Chinese physician, which is regarded as equivalent to a medical doctor in United States. There are as many Chinese acupuncture physicians as there are medical doctors in China.

Increasingly, acupuncture is complementing conventional therapies in the United States. Physicians may combine acupuncture and drugs to control surgery-related pain in their patients. It has been found that patients taking acupuncture tend to need less pain-killing drugs, and that surgery may heal more rapidly. Since so many studies proved conclusive, the FDA, after approving acupuncture as a valid pain control treatment, became involved by ascertaining certain controls. This included designing the manufacture of acupuncture needles for single usage only to avoid the spread of disease through poorly sterilized needles.

Before any alternative healing method can be considered valid, it is necessary that it undergo rigorous research by various scientific communities. This testing can be difficult to come by since the conventional medical field has a hands-off policy when it comes to medical cures outside their fields. Nevertheless, persistence has paid off, and now studies are conducted by some of the most unlikely sources, including those who initially showed antagonism toward any form of alternative healing. For instance, in 1998 NCCAM became dedicated to exploring complementary and alternative healing through a mandate created by the U.S. Congress that year. This includes the intermingling of rigorous modern science with cutting-edge healing modalities, and with those in the Complementary and Alternative Medicine (CAM) organization. Both NCCAM and CAM have since been supportive of acupuncture treatment for various physical problems.

As of March 2002, NCCAM supports sixteen specialty centers of research. Studies are being conducted by CAM for certain health problems. One center involved with research on acupuncture is the University of Maryland in Baltimore, where research is being conducted on alternative treatments for severe arthritis. Patients suffering from severe knee pain may consider acupuncture for treatment and thus avoid surgery. Such study is valuable for a couple of reasons: acupuncture is cost-effective, less dangerous, and unlike surgery, does not work against the body, but allows self-healing to take place. Another area being explored in acupuncture is its ability to help minimize hypertension. At the New England Research Institute and Massachusetts General Hospital, studies are being completed on the effects of acupuncture and its calming effect on patients. Patients undertaking this treatment claim that they felt as though they had just completed a meditation period. A sense of utopia was felt which remained with patients for several hours after their treatment. Obviously, such results can prove beneficial for those suffering from high blood pressure and various nervous disorders.

At the University of California, a pilot study showed that patients with heart failure had significant reduction in sympathetic nerve activation after taking acupuncture treatments. Consequently, these patients were depending less and less on heart drugs. The correlation between mind and body is most apparent in acupuncture, particularly in patients suffering depression. It is believed that acupuncture re-activates the endorphins in the brain and adds serotonin, which is sometimes referred to as "happy juice," and which pharmaceutical anti-depressive drugs are intended to mimic. However, like any drug, there are several negative side effects that can be neatly avoided by acupuncture.

IF YOU DECIDE UPON ACUPUNCTURE THERAPY

It is easier to find a licensed acupuncture practitioner than it once was, now that the FDA has approved it and some insurance plans accept this treatment. It has become a common treatment provided by more medical doctors and many chiropractors, some anesthesiologists, nutritionists, and even dentists are becoming trained in this field. There are now many web sites to search, and you can check to see whether they list the credentials and licenses of practitioners in your area.

To ensure a practitioner is competent, attempt to acquire some kind of referral or testimonies from previous patients. Usually those practicing in various medical or professional alternative-healing fields, since they are well established in the community, are a good place to start your search. For example, if one particular health individual does not practice acupuncture, they may refer you to one that does. Some purists have the idealistic belief that Chinese acupuncturists are superior; however, since most of them remain separated from the mainstream of the medical community rarely does a Chinese practitioner become involved with any form of research. Since, by Western standards, alternative healing is often considered experimental, this sometimes offends the Oriental doctor, who is well aware that acupuncture is far from experimental, having been practiced for thousands of years.

Again, it is pertinent that you seek treatment from a qualified practitioner. Some states are negligent in checking on the background of those involved with alternative medicine and some less experienced acupuncturists can get through the system without anyone noticing. The office must be clean, and needles never re-used. Usually the acupuncturist will open a new packet of needles in front of you to insure they are new. A well-experienced practitioner will avoid misplacing the hair-thin solid metal needles, thus avoiding leaving a bruise mark on your skin. You can learn more about meridian points, and where to insert the needles, by studying an acupuncture chart that is most often displayed in an acupuncturist's office. There must be fresh bedclothes to insure comfort and cleanliness, and good ventilation is essential since a session takes about half an hour to complete. Sometimes a heat lamp is used to keep the patient warm and to initiate better healing. To relax patients, soft music is played and the lights are dim; all in all, the experience can be a very pleasant one. Some patients feel energized after treatment, while others become deeply relaxed and even fall asleep. It is difficult to believe that one could fall asleep with a dozen needles inserted into the body, but with qualified acupuncturists, very little discomfort is felt during the treatment.

WORKOUT

The list below is a summary of the correct way to approach acupuncture treatment:

Make sure you check the practitioner's credentials. The acupuncturist must be certified and experienced and should be willing to discuss the procedure with the patient, what they can expect and experience during the procedure.

Find out before you start your treatments how many sessions you will need, and if there is a reduction in costs if you plan a large number of sessions.

Find out if the sessions will be covered by your medical insurance. While some insurance companies cover acupuncture, few practitioners want to bother with insurance paperwork, and may tell you they will file your claim but then you have to turn it in to the insurance company. Few insurance companies reimburse customers. If a practitioner is listed with the insurance companies, they will handle the insurance and you may not have to do anything except perhaps pay the co-payment, depending upon your insurance.

Make certain the treating room is clean, and new needles are used. In the past, the re-using of old needles caused the spreading of various diseases, including AIDS. When the FDA started to approve the use of acupuncture, the government insisted on practitioners taking precautions to prevent the spread of disease by using new needles with each patient. In addition, at one time acupuncture could be practiced anywhere and by anyone, which included some amateurs without licenses seeing their patients in some very dingy and disease-ridden areas. Now the health department has stepped in, thus insuring safe and sanitary conditions.

Make certain that acupuncture is beneficial for your particular problem. Some practitioners make claims that acupuncture can cure almost anything. Read up on this subject and find out for yourself the benefits of acupuncture. Under no conditions should you stop a medical treatment ordered by your family physician in expectation that you will be cured by acupuncture. This practice has its limitations, and you should know them. It is even best to discuss with your doctor if you plan to take acupuncture as a complementary treatment for what he or she is doing regarding your ailment.

However, you may discover that your doctor will deny the benefits of such treatment and may even become upset with you for partaking in something that is so experimental. In such a situation, you may attempt to persuade your doctor to accept alternative healing as a means of complementing your regular medical treatment. This can be achieved by showing him the latest information you may have seen, perhaps in your health magazine, or by having others who are involved with alternative medicine contact him. You can show your doctor some proof of the benefits of acupuncture. This may require a bit of persistency on your part, but results have shown that gradually more traditional medical doctors are starting to accept health practices outside their realm.

Make certain you feel comfortable with your health care provider and you are able to "freely express" yourself regarding your health concerns. Since this experience is probably new to you, and may even appear a bit strange, you need to be able to communicate and ask questions. Before you get involved with treatment, it is best to have a conference with the acupuncturists to see how compatible you feel about his suggested treatment. If you feel the individual refrains from discussing anything with you, you then need to look elsewhere for treatment.

Do not allow others to discourage you in your pursuit of alternative health care. You may be faced with ridicule and confronted by those who will warn you that you are wasting your time and money on such unproven therapies. If you do your homework, which is easier now since there is plenty of available data and the Internet, you will see that alternative medicine offers you a wide scope of natural healing solutions.

KEY POINTS TO REMEMBER

1—Chinese medicine sees humans as existing as microcosm entities within the universal macrocosm. Thus, principles that determine the flow of energy throughout the universe are applicable to the human energetic system.

The Chinese view the state of the universe as a dynamic equilibrium between polar opposites in nature, which is represented by their philosophy of yin and yang. The balance of yin and yang forces within the human body is critical in maintaining good health. When an individual is afflicted with illnesses, the subject of balance is very important to help the Chinese healer to determine the cause of illness.

2—Such disease-related imbalances in the major bodily organs can be determined by using diagnostic systems such as an AMI Machine, a computerized instrument that electrically measures and compares the terminal acupoints for each of the major paired meridians.

3—Chinese medicine seeks imbalance to be able to detect potential for illnesses before they occur. This enables the healer to ward off certain disturbing elements that may be responsible for beginning a disease. Electro-acupuncture technologies may allow us to measure subtle energy imbalances, which are precursors to illness. In addition, these same technologies can reveal illness in the physical body, which may already be present but which are still too subtle to be measured in conventional laboratory tests. The old adage that an "ounce of prevention is worth a pound of cure," applies here. Unfortunately, traditional healthcare tends to use the policy of waiting until an illness strikes before they take notice, which often can be too late. For example, consider the typical blood test: by the time a liver disease is detected, it is usually too late to cure it. However, taking preventative measures, such as avoiding alcohol, following a restrictive diet, getting regular exercise, and keeping your emotions in good balance, offers a well-rounded recipe for maintaining health.

CHAPTER 13

SPIRITUAL HEALING

It makes no difference how sick you are or
What ailments you are now suffering from.
If you have allowed yourself to be touched by faith,
you have allowed the healing miracles to manifest in you...

FAITH AND HEALING

The young man suddenly felt the tip of the arrow cut into his belly; he collapsed to the ground. The arrow seemed to come from nowhere, but the young man knew who his enemies were. From the type of arrow tip imbedded deeply in his chest, he knew it was from the Akia river tribe, who were vicious hunters. Struggling to get back on his feet, weakness overcame him. Tugging to release the spear from his bloody chest, he lacked the power to budge it and could feel life slowly draining from his body. The pain was unbearable and at that moment, he just wished the merciful Gods would let him die. As the young man started to slip into a coma, suddenly he felt a pair of strong arms picking him up and rushing him inside the straw and mud hut.

After administering healing potions onto the man's deep gash, the healing shaman chanted over the body all night. The man started to stir but then lay deathly still. As the chanting continued, the wounded man opened his eyes; the image of the healing shaman stood over him, his hands touching the man's wound as he chanted sweetly of the many purple skies, and orange moons the man was yet to see. His unyielding faith in the shaman's healing powers would sustain him throughout the night and the man then knew he would live.

The healing practice of Southwest American Indians included the sand painting ritual. The local spiritual healer carefully concocted and constructed the sand from an ancient recipe. After manifesting the sand, the spiritual healer placed the afflicted in the center of the brightly colored sand design that represented symbolic connotations. As the center of attention, surrounding this individual were his loved ones, who offered their healing wishes through their soothing soft repetitive chants as he enacted with the healer. During the ritual the healer introduced certain curing herbs that he had blessed, he also sang chants, while at the same time the shaman massaged and touched the patient. It is interesting to note, "touch healing" has become a popular mode in today's alternative healing.

The shaman's spiritual incantations are similar to the modern-day spiritual healing practices followed by the Christian faith as well as other religious followers. Proficient in utilizing herbal remedies, other healing means used by ancient shamans of tribal peoples included psychic powers. It was believed that calling upon certain healing spirits with whom the shaman communicated enabled him to receive certain messages as to the nature of his patient's illness and the correct healing process to use. To add, prior to any healing process taking place it was vital that the sick were first empowered with a deep sense of calmness of mind and spirit and had complete faith in their healer's skills in healing them.

To receive the most benefits of healing, patients had to undergo a period of preparation, as did the healer. To enhance his healing skills the shaman sequestered himself from all human encounter for a period of time. As a recluse, the shaman restrained himself from sex, food and drink, and spent his days devoted in ritualistic prayer, the careful gathering of the sacred healing herbs that he would use on the patient. The patient was prepared for the healing through prayer, ritual offerings and meditation and was permitted only to see close relatives.

Thus, we can see the afflicted were able to receive a variety of healing approaches, which encompassed the mind, body and spirit. This is comparable to methods used by contemporary alternative healers and unfortunately, ignored by our orthodox medical field. Actually, ancient methods of healing prove to be repulsive to many medical doctors since advances in medical science promoted cures that are more scientific. Our medical practitioners regard anything pertaining to natural healing as "unproven" methods of healing. Alas, the concept of healing from what nature had to offer gradually diminished into the stream of scientific discoveries; the test tube replaced nature.

Once science was able to wipe out some deadly epidemic diseases, it took the lead in the healing world. Natural healing techniques were antiquated by the medical establishment and believed to be practiced only by ignorant primitives. The "old wives' tale" that was based on many years of firsthand experiences of using various natural healing practices that actually "worked" became a subject of criticism, as was any mentioned of home remedies. In the meantime, today's alternative healing practitioners are utilizing many of these old healing methods, handed down throughout the generations. Medical doctors tend to scoff at any mention of these natural home remedies; however, an increasing amount of healers are becoming knowledgeable of the miraculous benefits of herbal cures and integrating them in their practice. Perhaps in the future, medicine herbal cures will completely replace pharmaceutical drugs. We can only hope.

In primitive societies, before the advent of modern medicine, they enacted the healing practices that their ancestors handed down to them through the ages. The village spiritual healer, referred to as the shaman, led healing chants, herbal cures, singing and dancing, healing sand paintings, methods of loosening the evil spirits from the sick body, a form of touch healing, etc. Belief was that sickness was the result of evil spirits taking over the body, thus, the shaman's duty was to get rid of them through his healing powers. As the spiritual leader of the community, as well as the medicine man, the shaman was an honorable leader and well trusted. The shaman's position, at times, could even be more powerful than the village chief. To add, where the latter's reverential position derived from political endeavors, it was through the skills of healing that the shaman gained his honorific position.

Earning the adoration of his people, he was the man of the people. He was empowered to intervene for the tribe by asking the gods to give special blessings when they were sick. The shaman's duties included acting as an herbalist, and with his expertise, he carefully collected and meticulously mixed all the healing potions used by the villagers. Each herb was chosen for individual illnesses, and was administered along with an assortment of symbolic enactments—dancing, singing, chanting, body movements, prayers, etc., all intended to facilitate the healing process.

Superstition played a vital role in the world of primitive medicine. Accusations could be made that the sick was guilty of some past deed, or that the patient's disruptive behavior amongst the villagers was the reason for his inability to get well. The tribe never blamed the shaman for his lack of healing skills. If conflict between a healer and a patient would arise, it was always the latter's fault. Those that were unable to recover from illnesses while under the shaman's care were believed to be "caught in the spell of evil forces," or perhaps were under the influence of enemies seeking revenge against them.

This part, in which a small rag doll is used as a vehicle of revenge, is similar to the practice of voodooism. The perpetrator inserts needles into the doll in order to attack his victim. Sometimes, the shaman decapitated the doll's head to mimic the occurrence in real life. Symbolic objects played a vital role. For example, the shaman had a collection of objects of all sorts, such as dried herbs, powdered bones, bits of hair, feathers, shells, rattles, miniature wooden figurines, etc., which were used for various means of healing. The shaman carried his array of tools in a sacred pouch, which always hung around his neck or waist. Thus, success of spiritual healing derives not only from superstition that is belief that transformation of some kind will manifest through mere belief that this will occur, but also what we refer to as faith. In "faith healing," belief that the healer is empowered with special healing skills has a powerful influence on a patient. This is particularly true with the healing practice "hands-on healing," where the practitioner has within his hands the powers to transform certain negativities into positive results. Just one magical touch in just the right place on a patient, along with a load of faith, has the power to heal. However, the responsibility of getting well is less on the healer's magical powers or even skills, but on the patient and the belief that the healing process will be effective.

FAITH AND THE POWER TO HEAL

It is evident that faith has the power to heal, and is a strong influencing factor over patients' health. As a member of the church's prayer team, I would receive many phone calls daily to pray for individuals requesting prayers for either a physical or emotional problem they were suffering from. One call was particularly depressing; it was a request to pray for a mother with four small children who was in the hospital with a brain tumor. I personally take these prayers seriously, even though I do not know who the prayer recipients are…nor do they know me. Healing requests are based on faith; faith that I will pray for them appears to be sufficient. Many Christian churches are involved with "faith healing," either via by phone or e-mail. Pathways Baptist Church, in Largo, holds three-hour healing prayer meetings each Thursday evening. In this time, prayer "warriors" answer a long list of prayers sent to them by phone or e-mail. It is an intense time, and can be trying because so many problems come into the prayer line, but for those who believe in the power of prayer and are involved with this activity, it is most satisfying to be able to spiritually help those in need. It is special when individuals give testimonies stating that this spiritual healing network has healed them, either physically or emotionally. Actually healing through prayer is a predominant practice among Christians, and virtually every church has its "prayer line" that members can contact when in need of healing. To activate the power of healing, those in need of a healing prayer will request that the entire congregation to pray for their healing or perhaps for the recovery of a loved one. Scientists are starting to believe that the power of healing may be enhanced when the number of those praying for the sick increases.

Many people believe that stories of faith healing, or any miraculous occurrences manifested through faith, are as ancient as the Bible, which regards Jesus as the central figure of such acts. Many passages in the Bible refer to Jesus as the healer by touch. Obviously, what was responsible for Jesus' miraculous healing, such as enabling the blind to see and the cripple to walk, was the belief that he had the power of healing (sic).

EMBRACING SPIRITUAL HEALING

As we shift from the materialistic, mechanistic, Newtonian world view to the Einsteinian, quantum mechanics, alternative medicine and the people who practice will be the basic predominant healing trend. Today's holistic view, which in reality has been with us for thousands of years, as it is embraced, such healing clinics will keep popping up all over the place. Some will practice various ancient healing ways, such as Ayurvedic healing, which entails taking into account nature and the vibration of the universe, as well as the introduction of American Indian herbal medicine and shamanism, magical and spiritual healing techniques, which consider the emotional and spiritual state of the sick.

This integrating physical with emotional and spiritual well-being is a holistic concept practiced for over two thousand years by the Essenes, who produced such healers as John the Baptist, John the Divine, and, of course, Jesus. This tradition reemerged around 1400s through the efforts of Constantine the African, who studied Essene texts in the Monte Cassino monastery and then taught them at the Salerno School of Medicine in Italy. Today, as always, there exist evolved healers who continue to carry on these harmonistic healing traditions that Dr. Richard Gerber, author of *Vibrational Medicine*, romanticized about and hoped for its return. This type of healing that these healers shared derived from their own harmony and love. It is a holism based not on the latest far-out diagnostic tool, or on one or two progressive healing approaches, but from the belief of the importance of being involved in every aspect of the healing. It is a simple and whole-person multi-level energetic approach, rather than a series of fragmented, alternative therapies.

Dr. Gerber claims, "A system of medicine which denies or ignores its existence (spirit) will be incomplete because it omits the most fundamental quality of human existence, the spiritual dimension." He points out and clarifies the concept of "Spiritual Nutrition and the Rainbow Diet." The idea is that "the tissues which compose our physical form are fed not only by oxygen, glucose, and chemical nutrients, but also by higher Vibrational Energies, which endow the physical form with the properties of life and creative expression." No doubt, living a harmonious lifestyle, taking into consideration and indeed nurturing the spiritual aspect of humans and integrating it with the healing processes is a vital means of healing. The ancient biblical healers knew this very well. Healing by prayer and through Christ's merciful touch reflects in the methods some holistic healers use today. For example, one particular modern healing method is called Reiki, which is based on "touch-healing" in combination with prayer.

KEY POINTS TO FOCUS ON

1—Illness may be a symbolic reflection of our own internal state of well-being such as feelings of conflict, unrest, spiritual blockage and imbalance, which can affect our physical well-being. Thus, we can become more vulnerable to external forces that attack our bodies. The chakras and energy meridians are affected by our emotions, and can become weakened when we experience stress, which ultimately results in a localized system breakdown in the physical body, i.e. disease.

2—Illness is an indication that we are constricting the natural flow of creative consciousness and subtle life-energies through our multidimensional body/mind/spirit complexes. Disease is a symbolic warning message that something has gone wrong within the system. We need to readjust the areas of imbalance in order to achieve good health.

3—When an individual experiences a blockage in working through some emotional or spiritual issue, it may result in a blocked flow of energy in the corresponding chakra, thus constricting the flow of life-energy to the associated bodily organ. Hence, within time, such blockage will express itself in illness.

4—Regarding the chakras, the heart chakra is the most basic point relating to our overall feeling of physical and emotional well-being. With spiritual enactments and through love, it can open like a fresh flower. The heart chakra is the passageway to good health.

THE HEALING OF MARY BAKER EDDY

Mary Baker Eddy, author of *Science and Health*, continues to be one of the influential researchers and authors on the subject of the mind, body and spirit. Born in 1821, she was way ahead of her times in the field of spiritual healing. Her book on spiritual healing which includes scriptures from the Bible has been the center for motivating readers to seek out spiritual healing rather than turning to orthodox healing.

Her research discovered that pain often manifests itself through one's belief that a particular incident will be painful. For example, a child falling, perhaps bruising his or her knee, will cry out with pain— often from the mere idea that the fall should result in a hurt. How often are children warned, "Don't run or you will fall and hurt yourself." Perhaps, charmed by a grandfather that the child is big and brave and that the fall is nothing, the child will believe so and come out of the incident unharmed. Pain often results from the belief that "there will be pain."

To add to the concept of "what I believe in—I become," a study was made of a selected group of college freshmen just entering college. Divided into two groups, the first group of students suffered anxiety and fear about entering college. The second group lacked this anxiety and looked forward to their future challenges. When studying these two groups, the first had twice as many occurrences of flus and colds as the second group. When delving further in this test, students in the more positive-thinking group explained their wellness in the lack of class-test anxieties, and considered themselves as having "good self-image." Above all, some of the total students relied on their Christian faith to nourish them in difficult times.

Ms. Eddy's research included how disease arises like other mental conditions, from association. She adds, since it is law of mortal minds that certain diseases are regarded as contagious, this law will obtain credit through association—calling upon the fear that creates the image of disease, and its consequences manifest in the body. This metaphysic fact shows itself in the following incident: An orderly informed a sick man that he had occupied the same bed as a man who had just died from cholera. Upon hearing this, the man immediately became sick with this disease and died. However, he had not died from cholera. After some investigation, it was discovered that the man who had cholera had not occupied the bed.

Unfortunately, considered non-viable, spiritual healing has no place in hospitals healing the sick. Furthermore, it is possible the role of "lifting up patients' spirits and offering them a sense of hope" could play a vital role in hospitals. However, since lacking any clinical connotations, at the present time, a patient is deprived of this healing concept. The only hint of spiritual occurrences taking place in any hospitals are in the chapels placed in some remote area where the bereaved can go to pray after a loved one has deceased.

LAYING ON OF HANDS

The use of "laying on of hands" for healing dates back thousands of years in human history. Ancient Egypt's practice of this form of healing can be read in the ancient Ebers Papyrus dated to 1552 BC. Four centuries before Christ, the Greeks used Therapeutic Touch therapy in their Asklepian temples for healing the sick. The writing of Aristophanes explained how he used laying on of hands in Athens to restore a blind man's sight and return fertility to a barren woman.

Included in the Bible, and known by every child who has undergone Sunday school classes, are the many healings Jesus accomplished by His "mere touch" on afflicted individuals. His miraculous laying on of hands, known throughout the world, and considered the work of the Christian ministry, was as vital as preaching and administering the sacraments. Jesus recognized that healing was more effective when His followers had total faith in His ability to heal.

The Pilgrim Center in Clearwater, Florida, a non-profit organization, is dedicated to healing the afflicted through spiritual prayer. Patients are brought into a semi-dark room, and two healing attendants inquire what they wish to be healed from and what holy personage do they wish to envision is in the room, such as Mother Mary, Jesus, God or any other spiritual figure. Then, the patients lies on a comfortable cot and the two women, with raised hands a few inches so as not to touch the body, chant spiritual healing prayers. The success of this healing session, running about an hour, depends upon the patient's level of spiritual beliefs and ability to receive these spiritual incantations. The deeper their beliefs, the better chance they will be healed.

WORKOUT

(The following are guidelines to help you better understand the processes of spiritual and faith healing.)

1—As with any form of alternative healing, check the practitioner's expertise and credentials, even if his or her approach is through spiritual healing. Claims of being a spiritual healer are easy because nothing decisive can be proven since this form of healing is a more current trend in the U.S., thus, little background is available on it. The best way to seek information is through references, word of mouth or the Internet, and testimonies of others who have been spiritually healed.

2—The environment in which you are receiving healing must be conducive to the healing process. It needs to be clean, quiet, and a soothing environment, such as dim lights (you do not want to have overhead fluorescent lighting) and soft soothing music.

3—Learn more about faith healing through the Internet and library. There are various ways to perform this healing. Find out which one you feel would work best for your health problem.

4—Most churches offer spiritual healing. If the church is small, usually the pastor will offer this service; however, in larger churches, various counselors or staff offer the service.

5—While laying on of ands may sound quite different than other healing processes you may have encountered, remember that the traditional medical field uses the concept of faith and belief when utilizing the placebo process on patients.

6—Try to develop a healing prayer group where members pray for each other's healing, perhaps outside the church, such as meeting in various homes.

7—Spiritual healing can take place anywhere. A group of individuals can direct prayer to the sick miles away. Thus, you can contact various churches and spiritual healing establishments and request they add you to their prayer list. Be prepared to pray for others. This reciprocal approach strengthens the power of prayer.

FRANZ ANTON MESMER

In 1778, a radical healer made claim that he could achieve remarkable therapeutic success without the need for patients' faith in Jesus' healing powers. His name was Franz Anton Mesmer. He claimed that the healing results, which he was able to obtain, came through the enlightened use of a universal energy which he referred to as fluidum. Mesmer claimed that fluidum was a subtle physical fluid that filled the universe and was the connecting medium between people and other living things, and between living organisms, the earth, and the heavenly bodies. His belief was that all living physical bodies, and even stones were impregnated with this life- giving magical fluid.

His research in Vienna included the discovery that illness could be cured by placing a magnet over afflicted areas of the body. His theory was that an ethereal fluid issuing from his own physical being created subtle healing effects in patients. In further research, Mesmer believed that this subtle energetic fluid was, in a way, associated with the nervous system, because he observed, they often caused involuntary muscle spasms and tremors. This healing can be equated with the Christian practice of touch healing, where a pastor touches a faithful believer on the forehead and the latter swoons to the floor; a practice called "slaying," often used in the Pentecostal faith.

Mesmer believed that when individuals were in a state of good health, they were in harmony with their environment, and with the basic law of nature, and if disharmony occurred...then disease would result. Mesmer came to the conclusion that the best source of universal force was the body itself, and felt the most powerful energetic flow derived from the palms of an individual's hands. A healer's hands, placed on a patient, caused energy to flow directly from healer to patient. Known as "magnetic passes," this form of healing became very popular. Unfortunately, from the mere suggestion, many scientists and orthodox medical doctors considered this method of healing to be a form of hypnotism and denied the relevancy of such healing. Scientists still refer to hypnosis as "mesmerism," thus, the origin of the term "mesmerized." Light has been shed over the years as to Mesmer's findings of the healing effects of laying on the hands. His work motivated further studies in this form of healing. Dr. Bernard Grad of McGill University of Montreal executed one of the most extensive studies on this healing method in the 1960s. Realizing the potential power of hands-on healing and psychic phenomena, as well as spiritual healing, he decided to look into it further and carried on with Mesmer's theories. He correlated the blind faith patients have with their healers to the placebo experiments used in the orthodox medical field. Both healing processes, while differing, rely on patients' total belief in their healers' abilities to heal them.

Regarding the placebo healing practice, where patients are unaware of the sugar pill they are given, they are able to acquire certain healing benefits, said Dr. Grad in his studies. His conclusion was that successful healing truly depended upon patients' faith in their healers, regardless of what mode of practice is used on them. In essence, it is the power of belief and the healer needs to focus and concentrate that belief so the recipients become thoroughly convinced of the healing powers of the healer.

SUMMARY

1—Try to recall when you prayed for someone, or for yourself, for any reason and write down in detail why you chose prayer and why you resorted to prayer.

2—Do you believe your prayers were answered?

3—Do you know of other resources you can turn to for spiritual healing?

4—Do you believe your present physical problem can be healed applying spiritual methods?

5—Do you believe that healing can occur beyond what you can see or even understand? Do you believe one's spiritual attitude affects one's health?

6—Are you prepared to receive the benefits of faith in any aspect of your life?

A well-known fable, which identifies with the miraculous works of Jesus, tells of a religious man caught in a flood. As the rising waters surround his house, he kneels in prayer, assured that the Lord will save him. As the water rose, he climbed on top of his roof, while continuing praying…calling out to the Lord to save him. Two men in a rowboat come to his aid. Declining their offer of help, the man cries out for the Lord to save him. As the waters continue to rise, a motorboat passes by with another offer of help. Again, the man cries out, "The Lord will save me." A National Guard helicopter finally flies over dropping a rope ladder. Now the waters have risen to the man's neck, but instead of panicking he calls, "The Lord will save me." Suddenly, the water submerges the man's head and he drowns. When reaching heaven, he questions the Lord. "Why did you not save me when you saw I was drowning? I had complete faith in you and you let me down."

"I did not let you down," thundered the Lord. "I sent you a rowboat. I then sent you a motorboat and then a helicopter. Why did you refuse their help?"

CHAPTER 14

THE MANY BENEFITS OF MEDITATION

He sat for hours in silence, nothing else did he care, seen all
Things in the world, but nothing could compare from
The deep darkest shadows he had reached the divine. Though
Meditation, he gradually reached the sublime.

People who reach a deep meditative state of mind describe it as "sublime."

This chapter is quite extensive because it covers a spectrum of healing meditations. To start, belief that long-term practice in meditation is beneficial to the whole human being—mind, body and spirit— thus resulting in the maintaining of all-around good health. Meditation is a healing practice bringing together all of these aspects of the human being, and with emphasis on maintaining emotional and physical balance.

CAN MEDITATION ACTUALLY SAVE LIVES?

Research has proven stress can kill, now let it be proven meditation can save lives. Dr. Arthur Aron of the University of California of Santa Cruz claims there is scientific evidence that meditation can prolong life. This impressive conclusion states that daily meditation practice lowers blood pressure, stress-related disease and improves mental functioning, which can curtail the onset of Alzheimer disease. Research at Harvard

University presented in the *Journal of Social Psychology* covers a study conducted with seventy-three volunteers with an average age of eighty-one, from eight homes for the elderly. These control environments enabled researchers to keep records over a period of time on those who were randomly assigned to practice Transcendental Meditation, which is called mindfulness training, or a simple relaxation program or no training at all. Those choosing meditation practiced consistently on a daily basis. Three years later, all twenty of those taught Transcendental Meditation were still alive. Survival rates in the other groups were seventy-seven percent and sixty-five percent. Hence, this study gave a sound indication of the benefits derived from practicing meditation. TM induces "a distinctively deep state of rest while the mind is alert but in a very settled quiet state" claims study co-author Charles Alexander. The volunteers practiced each meditative technique for twenty minutes, twice daily, during the twelve-week experiment. Alexander attributed the study's outcome to TM's combination of high wakefulness, which he said combats atrophy of the mind. He adds, "The deep wakeful restfulness releases stress from the nervous system." Levels of stress-related biochemicals such as adrenaline and cortisols dramatically decrease during a meditative state.

While traditional relaxation may be beneficial in relieving physical stress, it lacks the benefits of completely quieting the mind, which only meditation can do. In attempts to deal with mental conflicts, relaxation only offers a temporary period of escape. In the meantime, the psyche retains these conditions. The nervous system remains the same, because it has not been conditioned for the process of "complete mind inertia" during relaxation. The individual has not altered his or her attitude or come to terms with dealing with stress.

However, meditation offers more permanent and deeper psyche changes. Edward W. Maupin of the Neuropsychiatric Institute, UCLA Medical Center in Los Angeles, California, claims meditation promotes a sense of deeper personal resources, of solidity and strength, thus equipping one with beneficial characteristics in dealing with life's trials and tribulations. Meditation is first of all, a deep passivity, combined with awareness. While other forms of relaxation can help slow down the heart rate, they also cause mental and physical sluggishness, whereas meditation does the reverse. While it too promotes relaxation, its primary benefits are more potent, such as heightening awareness and sharpening the senses.

MEDITATION BENEFITS MIND, BODY SPIRIT

A well-tuned violin playing harmoniously, no discordance can cause it to play off key.

From ancient Eastern cultures to Native American Indians, meditation was a vital part of their lives. Used in healing rites and rituals, the medicine man, through meditation, communicated with the spirits, requesting them to bestow onto him psychic powers so the source of his patient's illness could be revealed to him. Gone are the spirits and shamans; today's modern techniques of meditation retain very little echo of their past. While ancient healing shamans have passed on, their healing magic seems to re-emerge in the various meditation techniques practiced in alternative healing. Meditation has always been to serve beneficial needs pertaining to mental and physical afflictions. Scientific studies are continuing to probe through new vital information regarding the merits of the practice of meditation as a healing factor.

MEDITATION AND BRAIN POWER

Since meditation nurtures concentration, it thus improves memory. Recently, the education field has recognized that meditation can assist students prone to test stress. Several students volunteered, prior to taking a test, to devote fifteen minutes to meditative exercise. The results, these students had higher test scores than those who did not participate. To add, this group claimed the relaxed euphoria they felt helped them enjoy the challenge of test taking. As for health benefits, they were obvious… the meditating students had lower heart rate and blood pressure during the test period than the stressed-out students.

Now we cannot expect traditionally minded schools to initiate students into sitting on the floor in the lotus position, in silent meditation, prior to taking an exam. However, with scientific reports promulgating the many benefits of meditation, it almost borders on the unethical not to introduce some form of meditation into the classroom to relieve students of test stress syndrome.

To support this concept, reports have indicated that stress hinders learning, thinking, and creativity. Several recent studies have proved that high blood pressure also leads to a decline in intelligence as measured by various IQ and performance tests. The cause of this decline in mental activity is related to a decrease in the supply of oxygen and other blood- carried nutrients to the brain due to the constriction of brain capillaries caused by the elevated blood pressure. Meditation alters the brain-wave activity. The high-frequency/low-amplitude beta waves of normal consciousness are transformed during meditation to the much lower frequency and higher amplitude alpha and theta waves. Studies reveal when your brain is working in these lower frequencies it is more powerful and potent, and is related to states of higher thinking, efficiency, enhanced creativity, and the improvement of cognizance skills, the latter being essential in flexible thinking. Thus, your mind is more receptive to outside information, and can quickly alter "what is needed," and then siphon out useless data. Such beneficial states enable your brain to continue to grow and evolve into "higher states of order" of complexities, thus become more effective.

MEDITATION PSYCHE-EMPOWERMENT

Another benefit discovered was that long periods of meditation help to develop the psyche's sensitivities. Reaching the "enlightenment" plateau helps one to become universally conscious, where all cosmos, all people appear as one. Modern sense of time and space holds no meaning. You sense "time" as being a cosmic ocean in eternity and space. The boundaries of individual life are not restricted to the boundaries of the body, and to one's family or one's immediate environment; they extend far beyond that sphere to the limitless horizons of cosmic life.

This expansiveness, derived from meditation, unfolds all potential for divineness, bringing consciousness to the high pedestal of god consciousness. Meditation can lift your life to a state of eternal freedom, supplementing it with unlimited creative energy. Less stimulation is needed to experience contentment, thus enabling one to experience increased satisfaction with less effort; experiences of gratification appease; life becomes enriched with a larger bounty of pleasures.

MEDITATION AND HEIGHTENING THE SENSES

There are five senses of perception and five organs of action. The senses of perception are sight, smell, hearing, taste and touch. The organs of action are hands, feet, tongue and the two organs of elimination. Through the five senses, the mind perceives, and through the five organs of action, it acts. For perception, the mind brings to bear upon the external world through the senses, and action brings to bear upon the world through the organs of action. These senses and organs become dull from lack of full use. Certain environmental conditions are responsible for diminishing the senses. The human psyche can self-will the senses to become dull for psychological reasons. Thus, for some, situations lose their intensiveness, and life appears less colorful. Disappointments and disillusionments can develop an attitude of cynicism, thus distorting one's outlook on life.

When the senses are saturated with the "bliss of being," the senses do not become slaves to passing states of the consciousness. Your mind, being satisfied, is not lured in wandering in search of increased excitement and happiness. Your experiences of external events become harmonious to your senses. When the eyes see a beautiful scene, the sight is pure, the vision is full; one is free from any malice or sinful perceptions. All is right on the level of perception, all is virtuous, and all is in the natural stream of evolution.

However, if the bliss of Being has not permeated the level of the senses, the senses are not in a state of contentment. The nature of the senses is to want to enjoy more. Often this need becomes an incessant search, which seems never to be fulfilled. During meditation, the finest sense of perception is unfolded, whereas, ordinarily, we tend to use only the gross levels of the senses. Tuning into one's most subtle and finest senses enables the whole range of the senses to become alive. One becomes more observant; things that had little meaning suddenly take on a fresh light. The result is an increased feeling of well-being with the least amount of effort on the part of the individual. While meditation expands experiences and revitalizes visions of things, you always remain in control. You are not lured by transitory situations in life but come to understand what is most precious. How can meditation have such power to alter one's consciousness? The answer can be found within the practicing of meditation. The basic answer, however, is that meditation develops contentment and peace of mind, and with these powerful tools, all things are possible.

In essence, meditation is a channel in which to experience and enjoy reality. It is not a means of escape, as some believe. Decreasing the mind's scattered non-logical thoughts, during meditation, enables the individual to focus more clearly on what is most important in developing mental, physical and spiritual self-empowerment.

The thought process involved with meditation can be described in the following: Thoughts evolve from the deepest level of consciousness. Coming from the bottom of a void, they rise as bubbles from the deepest part of the ocean. Gradually rising, thoughts become larger. A thought starts from the deepest level of consciousness, travels through the complete depth of the ocean of the mind and finally appears as conscious thought on the surface. Through meditation, these thoughts are kept stilled while in the depths of our consciousness, as the bottom of the ocean remains still while the ocean's surface is ever moving. In this state, you can become aware of the rising of the bubble of thought, and become conscious of its complete phase.

BODY POSITION FOR MEDITATION

The most traditional practice of meditation, adopted from the Far East from the sixth century B.C., is the sitting cross-legged (lotus) position, similar to the manner that the Buddha sits in contemplation. The Buddha, the spiritual deity of India, also called Gotama in his human life, gave up a life of comfort and riches to find salvation. For three days, Buddha meditated under the spiritual Bodhi tree, until he reached a state of enlightenment. Various body positions can be taken during meditation, but comfort is essential since meditation requires sitting still for a period of time. Some mediators choose to sit in the half-lotus position that consists of getting one foot on one thigh and crossing the other leg so that the foot touches the opposite buttock, similar to American Indian fashion. The meditator sits with back straight and head erect, the hands rest on the lap, or the hands can be positioned where the thumb and middle finger touch making a circle, suggesting the sun symbol.

During meditation, focus your eyes on a point a few feet ahead of the knees; it is not necessary to stare during meditation and keep your eyes open. Chauhuri, drawing on yoga practices, writes, "The radical approach begins with the resolve to do nothing, to think nothing, to make no effort of one's own, to relax completely and let go of one's mind and body; stepping out of the stream of ever-changing ideas and feelings, which your mind is, and watch the on-rush of the stream; refuse to be submerged in the current. Interpret the metaphor as, 'Watch your ideas, feelings and wishes fly freely. Just keep a watch. Don't let the birds carry you off into the clouds.'"

The sense of bliss arrived at after meditation enhances appreciation of life. What was once insignificant takes on new meaning, and that which appeared to be critical becomes meaningless. That is because, when the mind is relaxed, the psyche is more balanced; it works more rationally. Meditation is like looking into a clear pool, where everything becomes clear and visible. Thus, you are more able to discern negative trivia from more meaningful essentials in life.

ZEN MEDITATION

While numerous meditations relate to spiritual meanings, Zen, a sect deriving from Japan, is devoid of spiritual thought. This meditation practice's central purpose is the exemplification of discipline development. Its extreme exercises make it unappealing for Americans;

however, Zen's basic concept can be modified. The concept of Zen is the emptying of the mind, the ridding of all thoughts. Quieting the mind, keeping out all interfering thoughts is like the stillness of a lake devoid of ripples caused by disturbing breezes.

Zen masters have practiced this technique for generations. Its rigid drill-like techniques are tedious and only for those well trained. Under the guidance of the Zen master, mediators squat in "Yogi" position for hours without moving a muscle. A quick slap on the back from the sharp-eyed monitors keeps mediators from falling asleep.

Many meditation forms sprang from some form of spiritual concept, which served as a catalyst between a spiritual experience and deep relaxation. However, Zen meditation is primarily a discipline, thus is devoid of any spiritual significance. The basic purpose is to develop self- discipline and self-empowerment over the body, mind and spirit. In essence, when these three are balanced, good health is then insured. Meditation takes in the concept that illnesses occur when there is any type of imbalance; thus, through meditation, individuals can have more control over their illnesses and the lessons they need to learn in avoiding them. Through meditation, the soul may come to discover the true meaning behind the physical illness with which it is afflicted. If the person can correct that problematic emotional and spiritual dysfunction, the disease will often improve or completely abate.

Meditation has the power to cause unique changes in the body over a period time, which has been confirmed by various scientists. Itzhak Bentov, a longtime transcendental meditator, noticed how the body goes through changes, which occurred in heart and brain activity during a session of deep relaxation. These changes could be lasting. No one has to be told the health benefits derived when the rate of the heart is slowed down. When the body is relaxed, there is a well-balanced rhythmic, up- and-down pulsation of the body as measured on the ballistocardiograph. Meditation causes the entire body to slow down; the heart slows to a regular and well-pronounced beat.

WORKOUT

Start with breathing exercises, concentrating on inhaling and exhaling while counting to 100. If you lose concentration, tell your mind to be still. At first, you will find it difficult for your mind to empty its thoughts, because we have been taught to keep our minds active and equate an empty mind as an indication of weakness. With determination, eventually, your meditation will become easier, and you should start to discover a sensation of transformation in a few weeks.

Empty your mind by visualizing all your thoughts being released from an opening on top of your head. Clearly see this image, visualize these thoughts disappearing into the air. Make them disappear so they do not interrupt your meditation. If more thoughts fill your mind while meditating, quickly push them out as you did the when you started your meditation. The mind needs to be clear and not disrupted by mundane thoughts. Although these thoughts persistently develop, they can be controlled, which requires practice like any other skill. Eventually, maintaining a tranquil mental state becomes easier, and as the mind becomes more disciplined, slipping into meditation can become almost instant and interruptions become easier to ignore.

During meditation, the personality undergoes changes where one may appear withdrawn or distracted from life and daily problems, which some may interpret as aloofness. This is because when learning to avoid the insignificant, only the essential is focused on. A calmer reaction to stressful situations enables one to grasp onto the whole picture rather than focusing on details.

Meditation can easily be self-taught. The simplest technique to use in acquiring a deep meditative state is, each morning and before retiring at night takes a fifteen-minute break for meditation. Find a quiet area where there is minimal or no interruption and start your deep breathing relaxation steps. Sitting upright avoids falling asleep, and also enables the blood to flow evenly; whereas lying down inhibits oxygen from entering the brain, thus developing sluggishness. Morning meditation is beneficial for calming and preparing the psyche for the activities of the day, and it develops such beneficial tools as concentration and sharp awareness. Evening meditation helps you rid your body of the day's stresses and helps you relax so you can go to sleep faster and stay asleep longer. Meditation should be regarded as a sacred time; it is a period where one can retreat into a space separate from all others.

FLOTATION TANK

Another technique for relaxation is the floatation tank. Although this method makes use of modern technology, the manner in which they operate is relatively simple. Essentially, the tank, which is an enclosed chamber-like contraption, the size slightly larger than a person, acts like a protective womb. The sensation produced while in this device is like being unborn, yet, lying in the warm security of the womb, which contains a warm liquid. About eight hundred pounds of Epsom salt has been dissolved creating a solution so dense—far more buoyant than the Dead Sea or Great Salt Lake—that anyone lying in the water bobs up and down on the surface like a cork. The tank becomes like a dark womb when the door is closed. This darkness is pitch-black, unlike ordinary dark rooms, which has slight ambient light filtered through the dark. Not only is there absence of sight, but since the ears are plugged up, there is a total absence of external sounds, a condition so alien to our modern way of life. With this turning off both sight and sound, along with the warm water at body temperature, where there is no feeling of cold or warm, one cannot feel the surface of the water touching the skin, the boundaries of the body seem to dissolve. The result is a feeling of being suspended in a void, an experience like no other.

Releasing of the sense of gravity, as the tank's inventor stated, "alleviates the sense of being pulled down by gravity forces, which we experience in daily life." In this floating relaxed atmosphere, the tank uses technological means to quickly, easily, reliably and safely turn off the senses, now that is not needed in the meditative technique, such as concentration on breath, chanting, repetition of mantras, and other meditation practices. Similar to these other meditation techniques, periodic floats have been found to reduce heart rate, and levels of stress-related biochemicals in the bloodstream. Studies show that floating not only reduces this condition during the float period, but also keeps the levels low for days and in some cases weeks. An additional benefit is that blood vessels and capillaries are caused to relax and dilate, thus increasing the flow of blood to the brain tissue…nourishing brain cells.

CHAKRA MEDITATION

Far back, a thousand years ago, an exercise called "chakra meditation" was practiced by the ancient Hindus; its benefits are still recognized. The concept of this practice is that the body is a vessel for all human experiences; certain bodily techniques such as yogi exercises and chakra meditation regulate physical, mental and spiritual functions. The chakra meditation includes concentrating on chakra points, which are located vertically up the spine. Meditating on these sensitive areas of the spine includes visualizing symbolic images relating to individual chakra points. Since the spine is the nucleus of the human body, it controls the complete nervous system. Blockage of any chakra points is believed to be responsible for causing various ailments. Meditation helps to open up these points, thus releasing the underlining cause of various disturbances. The following is an outline of how chakra meditation works, and the benefits arrived when properly executed.

WORKOUT

(Chakra Workout)

Lie down in a relaxing position and meditate by visualizing the following points on the spine. Then slowly go up to the next point on the spine until you reach the top point located on the crown of the head, then reverse, going down the spine and repeating several times.

The first chakra, below the spine, is identified with the earth and is connected to the physical dimension. It is the most primitive chakra and governs adrenal responses such as flight or fight, and lower body functions. This visualized point is of an egg with a snake wrapped around it three times.

The second chakra is located at the sexual organs. It governs creativity, rebirth, and relationships and is located in the earthly or non-spiritual realm of the human psyche. Meditating on this point reveals one's potentials for creativity. It opens the awareness that the body is only a vessel, which is used as a means of relating to the physical plane. Through these meditations, this physical realm becomes transformed into the awareness of the true reality of a human being, which is the non- tangible spiritual plane. However, this inner-self realization is manifested through the tangible physical part of our self or the body, the vessel in which we use to relate on daily environmental conditions. The visualization of this point is of an empty space, or nothingness, which is the state the conscious mind is in during meditation.

The third chakra is located behind the naval and governs our sense of well-being. Some visualize this point as a sitting Buddha figure. Meditating on the naval, where the source of life entered your body, is the best center point for your well-being exercise. This chakra releases aggressive behavior, limiting the need to control and manipulate others and moderates the ego. Meditation on this chakra includes visualizing the ego as a huge deformed rock which is thrown into the sea. Ridding of this heavy rock indicates freeing the ego from its cumbersome weight. The visualization of this point is of the Buddha sitting in the lotus position in deep meditation.

The fourth chakra is sometimes visualized as a burning candle, and is located behind the heart. This is the center of love. Concentration on this point brings the consciousness to the center of the body. This chakra is in both the earthly and spiritual plane; when connected to the chakras below it relates more to physical part of the body—sex, and the body's functions. When related to the chakras above, it becomes transformed into a higher spiritual plane.

The fifth chakra is the throat chakra. It is like a receptacle receiving clear clean water. This point is the center of human expression, and meditation on it clears ambiguities, helps one to see and express their feelings and emotions. Since ancient times, in the orient, emphasis was placed on what was said and the tone of voice used. Ancient wisdom believed the power of words had the potential of having a lasting effect on one's feelings, thus the speech remained soft and only kind words were uttered.

The sixth chakra is located behind the center of the forehead. It governs the logical part of the brain. In its positive state, it is responsible for the feelings of being centered and well balanced. Some visualize this chakra point as a starry sky with a bright moon. Blockage of this chakra can be responsible for the individual retaining certain characteristics that keeps one from reaching the full capacity of self-growth. It also can cause suppression of the individual's ability to acquire the highest state of consciousness, which is in the next chakra.

The seventh chakra is the highest point that can be reached. It is considered to be the spiritual point of the individual. At this level, the pinnacle of self-realization can become manifested. Located on the crown of the head, it is visualized as a lotus blossom with petals widely opened; symbolizing one is ready to receive nirvana or total bliss. The ultimate goal of visualization of the crown chakra point is to initiate a spiritual essence that not only envelops the individual but raises his/her consciousness toward the outreaching of others to help them light the flame of enlightenment.

Once the individual's psyche rids itself of negativities, he or she can project into the realm of positive experiences. When the nervous system works harmoniously and in accordance with nature only that which is meaningful to human growth and enhancement of life is grasped onto, while that which is unworthy is negated. Gaining this clear awareness in life, we learn to act with greater integrity and responsibility, and from this, we can become self-empowered in leading a life that is fulfilled and worthy.

Meditation helps one to grasp onto the essence of the self. It helps to cultivate depth and profundity of living, the appreciation of living in its many expressions...and it is free!

CHAPTER 15

SEEKING THE FOUNTAIN OF YOUTH

Ah, if there was magic bullet
That kept us young
That kept our hair on our heads And our teeth in
our mouths. But good health at any age
Is like honey from the gods.

Some alternative health care individuals refer themselves to anti-aging practitioners; however, their methods are questioned by the American Medical Association because their results have yet to be substantiated by controlled studies. If this new breed of doctors prevails, a modern Renaissance can possibly arise in the medical field that is responsible for extending the mental, physical and sensory functioning of youth into old age.

Longevity is a very popular subject right now. Years ago, concerns were focused more on how young one looked, and now we are seeing a surge of interest in youthful appearance and how youthful one can look. That is not wise health. Medical doctors are looking into this expanding research and many are determined to find the fountain of youth and in a scientific manner through intensive medical research. Thus, many research articles on the subject have been published.

HOW AGING WORKS

The question is, can humans live forever, or for a much longer time than we do now? On the other hand, are we programmed to die on a certain schedule? Aging involves many factors. In the early 1900s, Dr. Alexis Carrel grew cells from a chicken heart in a nutrient solution for more than thirty years. The result of this work was that many biologists believed that cells were immortal if they continued to receive the essential nutrients essential for life and if their waste products were properly removed. In 1976, it was reported by Dr. Leonard Hayflick, in the *New England Journal of Medicine*, that cells were programmed to divide only a limited number of times. Apparently, cells have a cell division limit varying from tissue to tissue. For example, skin cells that divide daily have much more capability of division than brain cells; thus, tissue that was studied contained cells reported to be able to divide fifty times. After that, the cell would commit suicide (apoptosis) and die. Following Hayflick's work, many biologists could not believe Dr. Carrel's underlying chicken cells were actually immortal and that Carrel's study must have been flawed. They believed the heart cells continued to be viable because new cells were added to the culture each day with the nutrient solution. This solution was extracted from living chicken embryos that may have contained living cells that were inadvertently added to the culture medium.

Designed differently, after ten divisions, Hayflick subjected certain human cells to freezing temperatures. After being thawed out, he discovered the cells would remember they were capable of only dividing about forty times. The cells seem to know that they had the capability of dividing only about fifty times and then would die, thus proving that cells were not immortal but programmed to die after a specific number of divisions.

INCREASING OXYGEN FOR HEALTH

Some new research links increased oxygen to growing younger. We can live weeks without water, but only minutes without oxygen. Without oxygen we die.

For the past twenty-five years, Dr. Samuel West has been researching the critical need for sufficient oxygen. In his search, he has observed that the absence of sufficient oxygen can result in disease and death, and is a significant robber of the vitality of youth. His recent book, *The Golden Seven Plus One*, documents the complete healing of several major illnesses through oxygenation of the body. Dr. West's research has led to a scientific conclusion of how disease develops and how correct oxygenation can prevent and even reverse the disease and aging processes.

One mistaken notion in the medical field's understanding is that since oxygen is present in the air, we breathe enough of it to be taken in our bodies to remain healthy. However, present research conveys quite the reverse. When blood protein, poisons and water are released into the cells from the blood stream, it becomes impossible for the cells to take on oxygen. To start, enough oxygen is needed in the bloodstream to switch on the potassium pump in every cell. These sodium potassium pumps generate electricity in every living organism. When this electrical energy is working properly, our bodily functions work in a super-energetic manner. Dr. West has summarized in his study that one of the reasons why athletes are usually so healthy is because during their exercise their bodies require more oxygen. The consensus is that "the more oxygen taken into the body the healthier we are," and that shallow breathing, which most of us commonly do, causes all kinds of illnesses. Deep breathing activates the lymphatic vessels, which run alongside the blood vessels, as well as in between and through the cells that separate the blood and the lymphatic system. The lymphatic vessels are the conduits that pull out the poisons, dead cells and excess water to keep the cells in a dry state, which eliminates disease. Dr. West adds that poisons in our system can derive from experienced emotional reactions, from poor eating habits and from the environment. One of the first indications of someone suffering from a toxic reaction is the feeling of overwhelming thirst because the water being pulled out of the blood causes loss of energy.

Deprived of an adequate supply of oxygen, the body becomes more vulnerable to disease. Dr. Otto Warburg, winner of a Nobel Prize for physiology and medicine, concluded that oxygen deprivation was a major cause of cancer and that with a steady supply of oxygen to all the cells, cancer could be prevented indefinitely.

The question remains, if oxygen is so vital for good health, why are so many of us oxygen deprived? We have to breathe to exist; many of us are little concerned in how we breathe or what we breathe. No doubt, our polluted air and inactive lifestyles have much to do with the lack of healthy oxygen. In addition, poor diet, such as processed foods, lack oxygen and few are on a diet of raw food and vegetables, which are alive with oxygen.

This rapid aging effect of reduced oxygen is evident particularly with smokers. The odorless gas in cigarettes is 240 times stronger than oxygen in its magnetic attraction to hemoglobin, and when bonded to the blood cell it instantly eradicates the molecule of oxygen that was there. This results in oxygen deficiency, which in turn prevents the cellular absorption of nutrients. The cells in a smoker's body age quickly due to cell starvation. What is the answer to adequate oxygen absorption? To stay away from smoking, also deep breathing exercises, and consuming energy—raw fruits and vegetables— the latter should be dark leafy green vegetables such a spinach, turnip greens, broccoli, celery, sprouts, cabbage, and to add a daily regimen of exercise.

As we age, we become increasingly vulnerable to disease. There are two basic reasons for this: First, the body's ability to fight off viruses, bacteria and cancer cells declines with age, starting in adolescence. Second, the processes required for proper health maintenance of tissue function, such as the ability to metabolize sugar, handle cholesterol, and clear the kidneys of toxins become progressively less efficient.

EXERCISE FOR STAYING YOUNG WORKOUT

(Listed below is information on starting an exercise program.)

1—Look for a local gym, or perhaps at the YMCA, or your local recreation center. Usually these places are inexpensive, although they do not have the added luxuries that health spas have. You will find that some places offer unique exercises, as yoga, and the current popular exercise Pilates, along with the typical aerobics, for which you usually have to pay a small fee. If you are seeking luxury, then a health spa is for you. There you can be pampered with a swimming pool, sauna, and whirlpool, and of course, a gym loaded with all sorts of exercise equipment. You will need to be instructed on how to use the equipment; a good way to do so is have a personal trainer. A trainer will work out a particular exercise for you and will work "one to one" with you. These spas can be very expensive and usually an expensive membership is required. To add, lifting weights should be approached with caution, first lifting light weights, then learning exactly how they should be lifted. When signing up as a member, make certain you know what kind of contract you are getting. Lifetime memberships mean you do not have yearly dues, which can continually rise with no control over rates.

Fast-paced walking is excellent for many health factors, such as high blood pressure, diabetes, cholesterol, circulation, and releasing stress. Many recreational centers have walking clubs.

Jane, at age eighty-five is still active and vital. She maintains an enthusiasm for learning new things, which many feel seniors lack. Although she has some arthritis in her back, it does not stop her from performing her aerobics exercise three times a week. To add, her mental outlook on life is positive and she looks forward to many more years of living an active life.

Robert, forty, is suffering from various aliments including high blood pressure and diabetes. Working under stressful conditions as well as being a heavy smoker and drinker, his body is now suffering from this abuse. Alice, a ten-year-old, is overweight and gets little exercise. Suffering from diabetes, she has the body of an older person. While her playmates are active and involved with active sports, Alice sits home watching TV; she is constantly tired.

All three of these situations are related to lack of maintaining a certain healthy lifestyle, such as consumption of healthy foods, exercise, positive attitude in life and taking supplements.

It has been proven that keeping the body active is the best medicine for maintaining health, and this is true at any age. The Wellness Center located at the Palms of Largo in Florida is basically a gym; that is, it contains the standard exercise equipment as regular gyms do, and perhaps the weight machines are slightly lighter. The exercise facility caters to the residents at the Assistant Living Center and non-residents. The difference between the Assistant Living Center gym and other gyms is that the individuals attending come for therapy, and are accompanied by their physical therapists. Patients with various ailments, some quite serious, such as Parkinson disease, paraplegics, those suffering serious arthritis, fractures, or sprains, are going through an exercise regimen similar to those just exercising and not going through therapy. Of course, they approach their exercises differently; therapy patients use fewer weights and receive special physical therapy by their physical therapist.

The focus on the healing process is exercise. Therapists focus on strengthening patients' overall physical body rather than just on the afflicted area, and use every imaginable means to work the total body; stretching, bending, weight lifting, and even some yoga-type exercises. Patients referred to physical therapy when integrated within a gym setting have available to them an assortment of exercise modalities. No doubt, exercise strengthens patients and is responsible for hastening the overall healing process because exercise is excellent for the overall metabolism, strengthens all the organs (particularly the heart), the muscles, enhances circulation, and even is known to help Alzheimer patients because exercise enhances the blood flow to the brain.

There are two forms of exercise that are considered best for maintaining youthful energy and they are performed in two different ways: Aerobic exercise results in releasing certain hormones in the plasma for two hours, or even longer after you have stopped exercising. Resistance exercise, like weight training, causes spurts of growth hormone that stimulates IGF-1. While eating properly, mostly eating raw fruits and vegetables, it is believed that exercise is the best means of staying young and remaining free from ailments.

WORKOUT

Below is a guide for an exercise regimen. This includes running, race-walking, treadmill running and stationary bike.

1—Start at low intensity and slowly build up.

2—Exercise for thirty minutes.

3—Exercise three to six times weekly.

4—If you are forty or over and have been previously sedentary, aim for moderate intensity in the beginning. Once you have conditioned your body to the workout, you can try higher intensity levels of exercise.

Caution—Do not attempt to start any exercise program without first obtaining a comprehensive sports medicine physical by a knowledgeable physician.

WALK-JOG-RUN FOR STAYING YOUTHFUL

Two levels of running are excellent for maintaining youthful energy: First is running, which is the fastest means to lose body fat and change body composition in a more favorable direction. As the body gains lean body mass, it becomes more metabolically active. The second level, running to maintain the body's level of energy. Race-walking can be added to this category. It is very effective and does great things to the body, such as opening the microcirculation in the lungs—filling the body with more oxygen. Race-walking is also mentally exhilarating, a high calorie burner, and stimulates the mechanisms to detoxify the body.

Running guru Kenneth Cooper, MD, reports a study by his research group at the Copper Aerobic Center in Dallas, in which three groups of premenstrual women were trained to walk three miles a day, three days a week, for six months at various speeds. A fourth group was chosen that did not walk. The first group, which walked a modest twenty minutes per mile, increased their aerobic fitness by four percent; the second group, which walked a brisk fifteen-minute mile, raised their aerobic fitness by nine percent; and the third group which race-walked a twelve-minute mile jumped an astounding fourteen percent in aerobic fitness, more than triple that of the slowest walkers. Both weight loss and aerobic fitness are closely related; the faster you go, the more fuel you use, the better your heart and your metabolism respond.

TAKING IT STEP BY STEP

If you are overweight and over fifty years old, and perhaps just starting an exercise program, it is best to see your doctor and have a stress electrocardiogram. Anyone over sixty should have a cardiovascular screening as well as a stress EKG. Remember, you want to start slowly so you can continue to do your exercise at any age and without suffering pain. Walking is an excellent exercise for those who are unable to lift weights or have certain injuries. You get an added benefit from exercise that is done outdoors; it is a more relaxed environment than a gym and not as hectic or competitive.

Our running guru, Cooper, suggests the following steps for a beginner walker:

1—Purchase good walking shoes.

2—Attempt to find good sturdy ground to walk on so as to minimize possible tripping.

3—When walking, give your arms a full swing and alternate the swinging of your arms where they are raised to the level with your chest. This gives a good cardiovascular exercise.

4—Wear comfortable loose clothes that can easily absorb perspiration.

5—Carry a water bottle with you (you do not need extra baggage, such as a CD player, because you want to concentrate on your walking).

6—Keep track of your distance by measuring the mileage you expect to cover.

7—If you are going for a long walk, particularly at a fast pace, you need to do some warm-up exercises, such as bending and stretching.

8—Cool down by slowing down your walking pace for about five minutes, and then drink sixteen ounces of room-temperature water.

9—Start out walking a half hour a day, three to five times a week.

10—If you wish to start running, alternate fast-pace walking with a little running, then eventually increase your running time and decrease your walking time.

Lord Lee-Benner, head of the Institute of Aging Control and Nutritional Medicine in Newport Beach, California, claims the basic means of staying young is "peak immunity, peak mental function and a great body." Frustrated by his failure to deal with chronic diseases, Dr. Lee-Benner quit his job in "traditional medicine" as a consultant in psychiatry and neurology to do research for the causes of aging and disease.

Another doctor who left his practice to enter preventive health is Dr. Roy Lever from Washington, D.C., who made extensive studies in the past fifteen years pertaining to illnesses and lifestyle. He has devoted studies in preventive health, focusing on the concept that illnesses stem from lifestyle imbalance. He claims that some people readily catch minor chronic ailments, such as flus, colds, headaches, dysfunction of the digestive system, chronic fatigue, and numerous other disorders, as the result of depletion of the immune system. This depletion is directly linked to a number of causes of overt lifestyles, such as smoking, excessive work with minimal rest, stress, poor eating habits and lack of exercise, all of which are aging factors. Keeping young really means keeping healthy, and no magic pill will take off the years. Only a combination of good diet, exercise, taking the right supplements, and being involved with activities and having a good outlook on life can help you feel healthy and vital, and that is what being young is all about.

CHAPTER 16

FROM HERBAL SCIENCE TO MEDICAL SCIENCE

Over fifteen million species of plants exist on earth and two-thirds of them flourish in tropical rain forests. Much of these medical plants are being destroyed at an alarming rate by the encroachment of civilization. Over fifty species are being destroyed each year due to deforestation. As a spokesman from the Rain Forest Action Coalition stated, "The basic primary cause of this destruction is due to subsistence farming in Africa." While it may be difficult to put fault on people who are trying to survive, at the same time, the outcry against population growth raises all kinds of protests. While the trees are being butchered, the cornucopia of undergrowth is scraped out and burned and so are the many beneficial resources of medicinal treasures. In South America and Central America, greed is the basic underlying reason for deforestation. It is the raising of cattle in these now cleared wastelands, millions of acres of rainforest, to serve beef to fast-food and prepared-foods markets throughout the world, particularly in the USA, which is the largest importer of beef. If McDonald's fast-food restaurants were questioned about rainforest deforestation, they would not have an inkling of what was going on. South American cattle ranchers from the USA never have placed a foot on the soil of a tropical rainforest (after all they may get their expensive shoes dirty).

Another culprit of this deforestation is caused by wealthy logging companies for the making of furniture to toilet paper to toothpicks that are exported throughout the world. Hydroelectric dams, mining, and oil extraction are other reasons for raping this precious land. The question is where was the care and conscious concern of these intruders for the welfare of these indigenous people whose ancient traditions of life have been altered, if not destroyed forever. Obviously, greed speaks louder and clearer than concerns for human life.

Many who are dedicated to saving threatened rain forest species urgently carry out their commitment against all odds, but these plants are disappearing at an alarming pace and some lifesaving cures will never be discovered. It is interesting to note that the National Cancer Institute reports that seventy percent of the plants that have proven to be beneficial towards possible cancer cures are only available in rain forests. Now, collecting rain forest plants in the tiny Central American country of Belize, the American Cancer Society, whose ultra traditional background, never known to accept alternative healing methods, is turning to indigenous shamans or healing medicine men, who for decades have passed down their knowledge from generation to generation of the healing rain forest plants. These "wise ones" are being tracked down and questioned and their expertise is being seriously listened to and scrutinized.

RAINFOREST'S POWERFUL CURES

Today's orthodox medicine does not accept herbal remedies for healing…yet they should. Approximately seventy percent of today's supplements are derived from the plants in the fields; many have been used for millennia in the ancient healing systems. The drug digitalis, used as a heart stimulant, comes from the common foxglove (*Digitalis purpurea*). The Chinese have used it for 4,000 years. Digitoxin, the manmade pharmaceutical, is toxic as its name indicates, and is known to have negative side effects and must be used medically with great care. The foxglove herb has been used for thousand of years against heart disease. Quinine, derived from Cinchona bark, has been used for treating malaria for over 300 years. It was not until 1944 that anti-malarial drugs (quinine) were first synthesized in a laboratory. Some strains of malaria developed a resistance to the synthetic drug. In the 1960s, natural quinine was reinstated as the treatment of choice in certain cases.

Most recently, a new drug, Taxol, derived from the Pacific yew tree, has been showing great promise against cancer. The extract is so difficult to obtain, scientists have been trying to synthesize the active components. Long before the existence of one of the over-the-counter major pain relievers—aspirin—various part of the willow (*Salix*) were used for an anti-inflammatory agent and as a very effective painkiller. Years ago, scientists confirmed that the salicin derived from the willow family relieves pain, reduces inflammation and lowers fever. This was no news to herbalists who knew of its great properties and have been using it for decades. Willow bark, having another vital property, is used for rubbing on open wounds to prevent infection. Not until 1899 was salicylic acid synthesized as acetylsalicylic acid and aspirin, as we know it today, evolved on the market and took a while before it was used by the general public, who at that time were still using the willow bark from their own backyards. It was not until the mid 1930s before aspirin became a household medicine, that it was found in just about everyone's medicine cabinet; and to think, it all began from a steaming cup of healing tea brewed from the bark of the common willow tree.

Most of us have never heard of Nicole Maxwell, a brave pioneer and explorer who spent half her long life researching the dynamic healing properties of the wild plants of the upper Amazon. Nicole was a San Francisco debutante, and opera dancer in Paris during the 1920s and a wife of twelve years to a brigadier general. In 1945, she divorced and went to Bolivia to visit a friend, and remained there for twelve years. While hacking away in the jungles of Ecuador, she suffered a deep machete gash to her arm. Her guide, knowing what to do to repair the injury, obtained some dark and some red tree sap and gave it to her to drink. The bleeding stopped within a few minutes and the wound healed rapidly, leaving no scar. It was then that Ms. Maxwell knew she had finally found her life's work.

For the next forty years, she befriended the native Indians in the remotest regions of the upper Amazon, learning the secrets of the true treasures of the Amazon's healing life-enhancing plants. She became an ethnobotanist and wrote *Witch Doctor's Apprentice*. More of an adventure story than a medicinal manual, the book described a host of plants the Indians used to prevent tooth decay, decrease inflammation, painlessly extract teeth, dissolve kidney stones, heal burns and cure and/or prevent scores of other maladies. She eventually collected more than 350 plants used to treat more than 100 common ailments. She was confident that her work would be recognized by mainstream science, but her dream never came true. Medical science, being taken over by pharmaceutical companies, showed little interest in any form of natural healing, since herbs cannot be patented. Pharmaceutical drugs can only be patented from isolated healing constituents found within the plant. Years later, studies on the red sap that healed Nicole's badly cut arm revealed that the sap inhibited replication of the AIDS virus. This plant, Sanger de Drago, Spanish for dragon's blood *(Croton lechleri)*, contains ninety percent proanthocyanis by dry weight (ninety percent antioxidant.) An effort to isolate and market the active substance was abandoned when it was found its other constituents destroyed its therapeutic properties. This certainly reveals that nature knows what it is doing. Each plant has the exact mixture of various ingredients that makes each plant the most beneficial. Take away one of them and the healing qualities are less effective…if effective at all.

For the indigenous tribes trying to support their families in the encroaching modern twenty-first century, the rain forest has been more valuable to them dead than alive. Loggers, ranchers and miners have enticed the villagers with easy money and as a result, many tribes and forests have become lost.

At age eighty-three, Nicole Maxwell finally saw hope for her vision when she was introduced to John Easterling. Easterling was a successful importer of South American arts, crafts and crystal. "Amazon John," as the natives referred to him, had developed intimate friendships with the many tribes in his travels throughout the rain forest, which he visited over fifty times. John at the time had been cured by the local tribal healers, from the use of their herbal medicinal plants, for his hepatitis and Rocky Mountain spotted fever, a disease he had caught years earlier, which nearly cost him his life. His liver had become severely compromised, causing frequent dysentery. Parasites and Amazonian insects burrowing in his skin further challenged him. He had grown a great appreciation for the life-giving prosperities of rain forest plants, which saved his life. He grew to understand the urgent need to preserve these precious rain forest plants.

When Nicole invited John to join her, he gladly accepted to accompany her on her Peruvian jungles trip. At eighty-four, this fearless champion was to take her last jungle trek and John had the honor to be by her side. Fascinated by the mysteries and legends of the ancient Incas in Peru he had heard of since a boy, he had always dreamed of discovering the lost cities of gold in South America. Eventually, he settled in South America and opened a company called "Raiders of the Lost Ark," which sold pre- Columbian artifacts, such as handwoven textiles, recovered artifacts and handcrafts of the natives, then traveled to other areas selling precious gems.

One day, while in the Amazon Basin, he became very sick with recurring fever, sweats, and extreme weakness. He stumbled into a Shipibo Indian Village. The Shipibos, shocked at his deteriorating health, nursed him to health with their healing herbs. Drinking healing teas and making medicinal herbs over a period of ten days, John had completely recovered and even felt better than he ever had in his life. As he described, he became energized and felt full of vitality and also gratitude towards Mother Earth as he recognized the reference used by the Indians regarding anything which derived from nature. He realized that the many years he lived in South America, he had been surrounded by earth's healing powers and never recognized this fact until the healing shamans introduced it to him.

A few years later, after his travels with Nicole Maxwell in Peru, John decided to start a new life, sold his business to start a new business, and immersed himself into a different lifestyle. For over ten years, he has carefully imported thousands of kilos of carefully selected and documented herbs that were never irradiated or fumigated. He, with a team of international biochemists, medical doctors and naturopathic doctors, has ardently researched the plants of the Amazon that have been used for thousands and thousands of years by shamans and tribal healers. To retain all the healing goodness of the whole plant, the researchers have used an ancient process which extracts and preserves all of the bioenergetics and phytonutrients of the plant, including the trace minerals in the alkaline ash. This method, also referred to as plant alchemy, is much more costly and time-consuming and is used by only a few companies internationally.

A THRIVING BUSINESS

Today, John has a thriving business called the Amazon Herb Company, http://nirvana.amazonherb.net. His company uses only wild plants grown in virgin soils of the undisturbed Peruvian upper basin. All harvesting is wild crafted with virtually no ecological and environmental impact. The members of over nineteen indigenous tribal communities carefully and sustainably collect the herbs. For the first time, these villagers are feeling empowered and useful rather than just being exploited for the various richness of their forests such as the lumber trade, farming and mining of minerals. Once the valuable assets of the forest were discovered, the local inhabitants took on a new meaning of importance to the world for other reasons than exploitation of the forest's various wealth. They now had valuable healing herbs which they could get involved in harvesting for their own financial benefits. Since only the locals are aware of what plants are valuable, this puts them in charge of this venture, thus limiting outside dictatorship. Their homes are more valuable alive than dead. This leads to thoughts of discontinuing deforestation, where these precious herbs are to be found.

Our quality of life is being affected by degenerative disease. According to John Easterling, the cause is twofold. He claims the amount of toxins and pathogens in our environment is a major cause, along with the nutrient deficiency in our overly processed foods. Our organs and systems are literally starving to death. Throw in the toxins and boom and the result is extreme degenerative deficiencies. The information in plants growing wild in the Amazon is different from that in a tomato growing beside the interstate in California. The latter comes up from the ground in an artificial state, laden with a massive amount of exhaust fumes, which they suck up all day, year in and year out.

Certainly, the combination of the right nutrients and chemistry has been minimized, whereas those grown from the rich soils of the rain forest, in ecological harmony, far away from any form of toxins, have thousands of years of nutrients imbedded within, which are not threatened by toxic environments. John explains about "wild crafting," and adds that this method results in acquiring the strongest of the species because it is still in its original environment. When ingesting these herbs, we are also ingesting this environmental balance and harmony. This power and purity resides in us on a subtle level. John adds that when he goes up the Amazon River for several miles away from the towns and cities, such diseases as arthritis, diabetes or degenerative disease do not exist. John claims, "You are what you eat, so why not get food from the place of the highest concentration of life energy on the planet." He also mentions that the world has just begun to treasure the Amazonian botanicals. As Hippocrates, the father of medicine, stated, "Let thy foods be thy medicine."

Studies show that only three percent of over 200,000 Amazonian plants have been researched for their medicinal values. One of the plants, this herbalist claims, has comprehensive miraculous curative powers that are totally unknown to the medical field, which he feels is sad.* The herb called Phyllanthus, also called Quebra Piedra, which literally means "stone breaker," for ages was used to eliminate kidney and gallbladder stones and to clear out obstructions in the body. It is also believed to fortify the liver and gallbladder and used for the digestion system, and alleviating intestinal parasites. Its many multiple benefits include helping to cleanse the urinary tract and eliminate uric acid. In India, it is used for treating bronchitis, pneumonia and other pulmonary afflictions. Another plant, Iporuru (*Alchornis castaneifolia*) is well known to the indigenous people of South America for relieving joint pain, improving flexibility in movement and range of motion, for recovery of battle wounds and severe injuries. Iporuru is now becoming popular in America with our athletes; the herb supports muscles and joint structures and is known to have strong anti-inflammatory properties. Other plants are Marca for energy, longevity and fertility; Boldo to improve fat indigestion, Una De Gato to boost the immune system and Manaca to purify the blood.

For thousands of years, cultures throughout the world have known about the power of healing herbs that grow in the vast natural world. Ancient physicians, traditional healers, shamans, and sages have all utilized their particular remedies, oftentimes keeping them a secret from the world.

The intention of this information is not so much to focus on the tragedies of the rain forest but to offer information of the wide world of healing herbs which are found only in the rain forest. It is not the intention of this book to offer a wide span of information on herbal remedies because of the availability of that information in the many different books and fine magazines. Individuals can learn how to purchase good fresh herbs or even grow them yourself. The internet can give you that information at the speed of light. Also available is information on the properties of healing herbs, what herbs cure certain diseases and ailments, and how to correctly brew herbal teas and tinctures. Some people like the convenience of taking herbal pills and capsules; however, there is controversy over what method of taking herbs is the best. The consensus is that if you can grow your own herbs or find a local herbal grower that is the best way to go.

CHAPTER 17

THE OVERWEIGHT EPIDEMIC

FAT KIDS

Our latest urgent findings promulgated by the news media, which many of us already knew and didn't need to be warned, is Americans are getting fat. It is too easy to observe how the stylish bare midriffs come with protruding bellies. To make things dimmer, this overweight epidemic is affecting out children. Parents overeat, thus their children overeat. In Arkansas, over sixty percent of the adult population was reported to suffer obesity, and Kelly Brownell from the Yale Center for Eating and Weight Disorders claimed in *Time Magazine* that, **"This could be the first generation of American children to live shorter lives than their parents."** This statement should not to be taken lightly, since medical consensus is that underweight people tend to live longer than even those who are not overweight. What it boils down to is that much of the food consumed is not necessary for survival, and since our bodily mechanism such our digestive system is made up to intake food (ideally certain foods) intended for survival purposes. Extra food taken in the body is detrimental to the body's cells and organs; the body becomes overworked in its struggle to digest foods that do not belong in the system. To make matters worse, much of the American diet is unfit for consumption and never was intended to be part of the food chain for humans.

Tragically, in an age where modern science has promised longevity, our children may live shorter lives than their parents. Rather than having fit Americans leading our future generations, we may be faced with sick ones. Our children of today are the future of tomorrow; are we willing to accept generations of sick people?

Any physical breakdown affects every facet in one's life. Statistics claim overweight people are less productive, and suffer more ailments and have more absences from work. To add, as Americans grow unhealthier our health insurance rates will obviously have to increase. Medicare cost will skyrocket when the senior population is demanding at a younger age, all sorts of medical benefits for their sick bodies. Due to poor health, our future population could be classified as being seniors at a younger age and it is getting to that stage now. Women under the age of forty are getting diseases usually associated with older women, such as heart disease, diabetes, elevated cholesterol and breast cancer and often, this age group can't afford health insurance. Now, these diseases are spreading to our children.

THIS MAY BE THE FIRST TIME IN HISTORY THAT PARENTS OUTLIVE THEIR CHILDREN.

Now, there is the diabetes epidemic. Hillary Carroll knew something was wrong. She had spent Memorial Day happily frolicking in her grandmother's swimming pool. By evening, she was in terrible pain every time she went to the bathroom. Her mother thought it might be from an infection and the next day took Hillary, then ten years old, to the pediatrician. Rather than getting a prescription for an antibiotic, the one for a 220-pound person, the youngster was immediately admitted to the hospital. Lab tests showed that she had something far more serious—Type 2 diabetes.

Hillary is not the only overweight child to discover she suffers from this form of diabetes, a chronic metabolic disorder that, at one time, used to be called adult onset but was renamed in part because so many kids Hillary's age were getting it. As doctors have repeatedly warned, the U.S. is experiencing a diabetes epidemic. Some 18 million Americans suffer from one form or another, with 1.3 million new cases diagnosed last year—up from 878,000 in 1997. Although Type 2 diabetes still tends to strike people in their fifth or sixth decade, more children are getting it, a fact of grave concern to health officials. A statewide survey shows that middle-age schoolchildren eat poorly, do not exercise and have weight worries. Statistics show that twenty-six percent drink two or more sodas a day, fifty percent ate fast food at least twice a week, seventy-six percent have a TV in their bedroom, and forty-two percent were attempting to lose weight. To cut costs, many schools are eliminating their physical education programs and without exercise, our children will become even more overweight. Dr. John O. Agwunobi, secretary of the Florida Department of Health, remarked regarding the amount of overweight kids, "It just blows me away every time I see the numbers." What bothers Agwunobi most is the high number of adolescents reporting unhealthy habits at home. More than seventy-six percent of teens reported having a TV in their bedroom and seventy-eight percent said they watched TV, played video games or used a computer at least three hours on an average school day. "That's sedentary living, by its definition," Agwunobi said. "This clearly has major implications for the ways we're bringing up and nurturing our children in the home."

Dr. Zachariah P. Zachariah, a Broward County cardiologist and top Republican fundraiser, will chair a new task force that will look into this issue. He claims that the vast majority of his patients do not exercise and are obese…they are raising inactive children. Dr. Zachariah, along with Agwunobi and others, talks about adding more health education, slimming down lunch menus and increasing health physical education. The function of the task force is to find a way to motivate people to change their lifestyles. President Bush talked to experts and they agree that there needs to be a way to get the public's attention to start campaigns that will influence exercising and eating healthier diets.

Another pediatrician from All Children's Hospital in St. Petersburg, Dr. Frank Diamond, claims that more and more of his young patients are arriving with adult problems such as high blood pressure, high cholesterol and Type 2 diabetes. He claims by the time a teen is overweight, you have an overweight adult. He adds that this massive problem requires a public health and a community response. Others take the same attitude as Dr. Jim Gills, an eye surgeon and owner of the

Ironman Triathlon who stresses that the task force President Bush is talking about forming should stress physical fitness.

Some individuals working on this program agree that to prepare our children to survive in the future, concerns regarding health also needs to be addressed. Success does not come easy for those who have to spend a lifetime battling with various health afflictions. The alarming fact is that the young will be old before their time. Faced with so many challenges in a difficult world, such as exposure change, living in toxic environments, coping with pesticides in foods and chemicals in our water, and fighting daily stress due to overweight, kids face the added load of suffering health problems at a younger age. This is one health factor that can readily be remedied by self-imposed diets and yet still so many of the young suffer obesity.

No doubt, we are a nation of consumption and extremes, as well as consciously or subconsciously becoming immersed in measures of self-destruction. We overuse energy (gas-guzzling autos and freezing public buildings) even though not too far in the past, a whole city experienced a total blackout. Few people remember the horrific experience of waiting in long lines, several blocks long, at gas stations and with the awareness that the gas station may run out of gas at any time. It was then that the clever planning of commuting took effect, where responsible individuals rode together to work and play in order to save on gas. Not so anymore; we need to do our own thing in our own vehicle and the bigger it is, the better. Many fail to consider that their actions today will have an effect on the future of our planet; along with these other factors, overweight has the most direct potential of self-destruction, and that is a concern we should focus on.

DOING SOMETHING ABOUT IT

Obesity in children is a concern that got Arkansas involved. The state reported that over a quarter of high school students are overweight or at "risk." The state health director estimates that Type 2 diabetes, formerly known as the adult-onset variety, is up 800 percent in kids over the past decade. He reported that "This problem is becoming epidemic even with the middle and preschool children where over ten percent are overweight. Over-chubby kids are no longer considered cute, but sickly. There is nothing adorable about rolls of fat. Our youngsters are growing up with the type of eating habits that will follow them for the rest of their lives if they do not become knowledgeable about their eating habits."

The consensus stated that something has to be done about our obese children. The reason it took so long to come to this conclusion is that politics runs slow, too many involved do not give a hoot about the kids' health…after all, kids cannot vote. Who really looks out for the welfare of our children? Many working mothers are too busy to feed their kids properly, or even to bother to look at what their kids are eating away from home. The average instant frozen dinner, which Americans rely on so much, has over 1500 calories a meal and nothing much else; the foods served at fast food restaurants are even worse. Over-stuffed useless calories exist in the average school cafeterias where the basic menu is starch over starch and super fat mingled with super fat.

The state of Mississippi also took action. When the state's 1,139 public schools opened their doors for a new year, they tackled a new task, one they never dreamed they would ever have to, and that is to tell kids to eat right. Needless to say, that was always the parents' dedicated duty. Well, that responsibility is being shared by the schools, and in some communities the schools takes full responsibility. For the first time, schools will be asked to issue each student a health report card in the form of body mass index, BMI, a plan formulated by the lawmakers, then passed by the Briggs-sponsored bill. In other words, schools were to literally add a section to report cards, along with the traditional assessments in reading, writing and arithmetic; the measurements of a child's body.

Concerns have risen that making a child's weight public on a report card can stigmatize that child for the rest of his or her life. The state PTA president, Kathy McFetridge, claims that children tend to pass their reports cards around and with the tendencies of easily making fun of the other's score, this would just throw in more fuel to the fire and overweight people could just be constantly tormented. On the other side of the coin, it may be an incentive for that child to watch his or her diet.

Often, obesity is not the child's fault if the parents are not knowledgeable or conscious of what foods are offered at mealtime.

There is another problem, and that is, poorer families cannot afford the more expensive foods like fruits, vegetables or lean meats, thus starch is the staple of their diets because it is cheaper and there are those who warn that if you criticize children's weight problems, you could be criticizing their family culture. These warnings lead most people to believe that pasta-eating Italians and rice-and-bean-eating Hispanics are all overweight. To help alleviate possible harassment amongst children, Arkansas' new health advisory committee voted to modify the way they approach the problem. Health reports will be mailed out separately to parents and parents may even opt out of the program.

While Arkansas is the first state to embrace the health-care approach, similar policies are being explored in other states and seeking possible other means of approaching child obesity. Some drastic statistics are responsible for this growing concern; nationwide, fifteen percent of children ages five to nineteen are considered overweight, which is triple the rate twenty years ago. Pediatricians claim that obese children grow up to be obese adults. The reason, they are used to overeating and become accustomed to the type of food that is high in calories and fats. They concluded that these children face higher rates of hypertension, and various other physical illnesses. Kelly Brownell, director of Yale University Center for Eating and Weight Disorders, claims, "These kids are candidates for coronary by-pass in their twenties and ever sadder is the fact that this could be the first generation of American children that live shorter lives than their parents."

While the medical community has been making all sorts of noise regarding this issue, not much has been done to initiate some type of statewide plan regarding weight control for children. One move, however, was made by the American Academy of Pediatrics (AAP), which included a recommendation to doctors to make BMI assessments a routine part of annual physicals. In this way, parents are apt to take the problem more seriously if the overweight report comes from a doctor's office. Children are apt to be less offended if their doctor makes the report rather than the school, where other critical children can easily inflict damage on an overweight child's ego. People argue that school lunches and gym periods need to focus more on the health and fitness of the child and be forced to make the necessary changes. For years, there has been the controversy over poor school lunches and not enough P.E. classes, to which the answer has always been the same, "There just isn't enough money in the school system to accommodate such issues." The overweight epidemic has been addressed by New York City and California; they decided on reacting in a more humane manner than Arkansas and Mississippi in helping with the overweight epidemic. They quietly, but firmly, passed the law where schools no longer are permitted to have soft drink or candy machines and are making an effort to have better school lunches. This was quite a difficult discussion to make, since canteen machines bring in high revenue to the state.

The latest media announcement that America has one of the highest rates of obese children in the world is alarming. The movement towards removing soda machines from schools is just the tip of the iceberg. Soda pop is not the only offender; it is what children consume in fats, sugars and milks (from candies) and these poisons fill the vending machines in even public and private schools. It is obvious the subject needs to go right to the "heart" of parents to take a more responsible role regarding their children's diets. It is very clear that we cannot depend on greedy school officials, greedy doctors or greedy government officials to care for our children's health and well-being; they are literally killing our children. Take a stand and demand that our children not be fed killer foods in the school cafeterias and health foods replace junk foods in the vending machines.

At a time when schools are increasingly taking on responsibilities once left to parents, such as warnings against smoking, sexual behavior, dress codes, etc., it appears motivating children to eat properly and exercise has not made the list, at least for most schools. Still there is controversy that feeding a child is a parent's most elemental duty. For some, the idea of a school intruding in such an intimate issue by issuing failing grades due to overweight was horrifying. On the other hand, many agreed something drastic has to be done because of the lack of parents recognizing this growing problem. Of course, the simplest solution is through teaching. Workshops and seminars on health and diet should be offered by the government to those unable to pay for such training. For those unable to attend classes, health information could be sent out to households in which doctors have reported cases of overweight children. Parents need to be motivated to change their health habits and take the time to prepare healthy meals. Too many children today live off fast foods, which are fatty and empty of nutrition.

One notion regarding overeating is the kind of food children eat and how they are eating. The foods lack a "sense of satisfaction"; hence, more food needs to be consumed to attain that degree of satisfaction. Not too long ago, a case came in court where a desperate boy, demanding his mother make a home-cooked meal rather than getting something out of the freezer, raised the eyebrow on neglect and the unfit meals our children are being forced to consume. The judge took the mother's side saying that a busy working mother did not have time to cook; therefore resorting to a frozen dinner was acceptable. Obviously, for this boy it was not. Perhaps all day he faced hostility and cold indifference as many children do, where many parents have little time for their children. This boy was just pleading for a little of his mother's time and care and perhaps had nothing to do with what he ate.

Feeding is an act of nurturing, and for animals is a vital nurturing act; parents feeding their children is an act of love and caring. Too often, children are fed by some fast food establishment or eating alone without their families. Psychologists say that children are comforted by the home- cooked meal, where the family sits together at the dining room table; mealtimes become a psychological and social act and not just a time to consume food.

PRIVACY ACT

Obviously, there will be repercussions, the typical protest of interference with family privacy and rights, if this act manifests into a predominant issue throughout other states and the notion that if parents can't take proper care of their children, then their benefactors need to be the state to look out for their welfare. Perhaps this state welfare concern can be carried over to those households were children suffering bronchitis, allergies, and chronic sinus problems are being exposed to secondhand smoke. At a time when Congress is attempting to ward off kids from getting into the habit, and reprimanding cigarette companies to refrain from advertising to children, is it not the time to take notice that children brought up with secondhand smoke are more apt to be smokers when they grow up? If we are concerned about the health and welfare of our children, then this should be considered a pertinent factor in anybody's book. With these preventive acts, children can grow up without having to rely, the rest of their lives, on doctors and medicine to remain healthy.

Obviously, overeating is an indication of imbalance and in a world of many imbalances; it is understandable we are now a nation of overweight people. Many children as well as adults suffer from lack of discipline. With the need for instant gratification, whatever one wishes to do is acceptable, and the sense of moderation nonexistent, absurd eating habits seem to be the outcome. Overeating needs to be seen as a possible social-mental disorder and considered a serious imbalance problem. Individuals suffering from this disorder needs to evaluate their complete lifestyle, observe what they feel is missing in their lives, what may be disturbing them, why they may be feeling a sense of discontentment, which they may be substituting for overeating. This self-evaluation needs to be done in a constructive manner so that individual situations can be managed or treated by professionals.

WORKOUT

(Listed below are self-evaluation questions for those who may suffer from obesity.)

You need to ascertain what situations in your life you feel you may need a professional's help.

1—What do you feel is the major disturbance in your life at the present time?
2—Do you eat when you feel lonely, depressed or anxious?
3—Do you enjoy the foods you eat or just overeat by habit?
4—Do you consume food without thinking of calorie intake?
5—Do your family and friends overeat?

You probably know by now the many types of weight loss schemes offered, and of course discovered they just do not work. Diet control requires discipline and thought, and needs to come from the individual struggling with obesity. If you are someone suffering from overweight, you need to think of the sad consequences, which have been extensively covered in this chapter. Overweight is a disease, and the bottom line is that overeating is an addiction, just like any other act that is out of control. It is a sense of imbalance of the emotions, and until this balance is in good working order, no diet in the world will prove effective.

CHAPTER 18

THE SELF-HEALING BODY

Why is it we fix our cars, fix our houses, build bridges and towers, but never learned to fix ourselves.

Fear of disease can become a heavy burden on the mind but rarely do we consider that many ailments are self-induced, just as healing is self- controlled. Those who overindulge in food, alcohol, and other destructive lifestyles are directing themselves to negative results. Their health is in their hands. When the blood rushes madly through the veins or languidly creeps along its frozen channels, we refer to these conditions as diseases. It is the state of our mind that causes these two physical occurrences. When mental thoughts become harmonious, the blood flows through the system in a natural healthy manner; the mind can cause a disease as well as heal.

As the writer/researcher Mary Baker Eddy states, "Disease originates in the mind before it becomes manifest in the body." Chills and heat are often the form in which fever manifests itself. If the mental state is charged up into a positive mode, the chills and fever can disappear. A study with freshman college students discovered that those who allowed themselves to be mentally exhausted, depressed, worried, all deriving from the mind-attitude-belief system, and nothing to do with physical aliments such as viruses, germs, diseases, environmental conditions were more apt to catch the flu than those who had more relaxed natures and confidence in themselves. Those who have confirmed they are incapable of getting sick, that they just have too much to accomplish and are busy community members, contributing to various organizations, tend to live out their will. On the other hand, those who just know they have a weak constitution will live that belief as well. Perhaps the healthiest people are those who are in love and those on vacation. Obviously, this is proof that emotions, which *we have control over*, play a leading role in maintaining health; thus love, joy, faith and self-belief are controlling factors. Treating the core of most illnesses is by first attempting to prevent them. Alternative healers first prescribe a vast variety of vitamins and other key nutrients, as well as a regime of exercise and also to learn to recognize what the body needs and is lacking. Some biologists today are proposing that physicians take heed when treating patients in recognizing the body's valiant efforts to heal itself and take into consideration the body's miraculous ability to heal itself. Many physicians automatically prescribe aspirin, or a similar painkiller, to patients suffering from a cold or flu but an evolutionary reasoning reveals that such a therapy may backfire.

Beyond easing a patient's discomfort, aspirin also lowers fever. Scientists have discovered that while extremely high fevers are harmful to the body, a moderate fever is among the most powerful tools in the body's defense repertory. The activity of the body's warrior white blood cells becomes stimulated from a higher temperature, allowing them to race to the site of an infection more rapidly and consume microbes more readily. A fever also works phenomenally in inhibiting. The body has an enormous capacity to heal itself if it is allowed to do so. Unless extreme external negative forces continually cause disturbances, the body's DNA system has the mechanism to self-repair. That is the approach alternative medicine takes, whereas traditional medicine attempts to heal by denying the body's natural forces by healing with artificial means, which usually is temporary healing at best. This healing process discounts the body as having the capacity to heal itself, and relies on unnatural means of healing. It denies that healing is an inherent capacity of life and that DNA has within it all the information needed to manufacture enzymes to repair itself.

THE CHANGING BODY

The human body has evolved for millions of years. Throughout these years of experience, it matured according to its survival needs. As the environment changed so did the needs of humans. The phenomenal manifestation of the modern human being is a product of long-term experiences of cause and effect, of survival needs and the best means of staying healthy. An example of how one organ changed throughout the years are the eyes. Early man's vision was excellent because it needed to be relied on for survival. If the hunter's vision was impaired, he could not hunt. Now the eyes have different uses, and basically do not rely on sharpness of vision for survival. Yes, humans do have to see; however, they can still survive with impaired vision. Using our eyes quite differently than our very early ancestors has in many cases resulted in causing impaired vision. Actually, in our technology age, where the use of computers and TV viewing is so predominant, children are increasingly suffering from impaired vision, and it is getting more common to see them wearing glasses. In our computer age, eyes are used more for close- up details, which ultimately has a detrimental effect on the eyes, whereas our ancestors focused more outward (for hunting and farming).

As humans, their heads became smaller, and brains larger, they grew taller, and arms became shorter, feet and hands grew a few inches smaller, all due to the changes in our environment. The point is that nature took care of man's needs as his environment altered. When science came into the picture, the attitude was that now science knew better than nature and in its egoistical manner started to play the role of God.

The natural order of things is that the healing system operates continuously and is always prepared to aid in any illness. When an overwhelming illness occurs, the best means of healing is through the body's own healing capacity. Illness is part of the natural order of things; therefore, it needs to be approached through the manifestation of the natural order of things, since human beings are part of the natural order of life. As part of the animal family, our illnesses can closely simulate those of primates. Chimpanzee catch colds, suffer from arthritis as they age, and poor eyesight. They also can have disruptive digestive systems, and like us, even suffer from depression. Scientists, particularly Jane Goodall, have for many years studied chimpanzees and observed their behavior during illnesses and how they went about healing themselves, such as their diet and their behavior. Goodall noticed that a sick chimp was very careful what it ate, very carefully scrutinizing each fruit consumed. Obviously, diet, particularly during illness, was keenly observed and certain herbs would be dug up and consumed. A sick chimp sometimes got particular attention from the group through special grooming, as though the touch and care added to the chimp's healing.

When humans' healing power is interrupted by unnatural means, their power of self-healing weakens. The healing system has its own diagnostic capability and can recognize damage. It can remove damaged structure and replace it with normal structure. It not only acts to neutralize the effects of serious injury (as in the SOS response in *E. coli*), it also directs the ordinary moment-to-moment corrections that maintain normal structure and function (as in the proofreading and editing activity of DNA polymerase 1). Healing is natural; it arises from the internal structure of DNA.

SELF-HEALING OF A WOUND

A good example of natural self-healing can be seen in the process of wound healing. A finger cut with a knife initially causes pain; it is the body warning that damage occurred. If this pain did not occur, the cut may go unnoticed, thus the special attention need to heal it would go unnoticed. It is this very factor that concerns diabetic patients. Often this disease causes uropathy to occur in the feet; they become numb. If injured, the individual cannot feel the damage due to the numbness. Similar to a baby's cry for milk, the natural cry acts like an alarm for attention to get food. In very poor third world continues, many babies do not cry for milk because they know there will be no response.

As for the cut finger, the pain subsides quickly; it is how you perceive the activity of peripheral nerves notifying your brain of the injury.

Unless there is a blood-clotting disorder, the bleeding from the cut will also stop shortly with the formation of a clot that will harden to a protective scale. Then there is a slight inflammation around the edges of the wound. This is an immune response resulting from the migration of white blood cells to the area to defend against the entrance of germs and to clear the damaged area of dead and dying cells. This is followed by cells growing out from the edges under the clot which fuse in the midline forming what is called new skin. This is followed by a formation of a grainy tissue called granulation tissue, which eventually fills the space of the wound. Finally, the immune cells recede, new skin develops and thickens and the cut is completely healed. All this is done by the body's own healing mechanism. Obviously, if the cut was deeper, the body's natural healing power may not have been able to heal the wound, but it can play a strong part in the healing process. Healthy individuals can expect healing more rapidly than those with weaker immune systems.

Such steps in wound healing can be seen in the repair of a simple bone fracture. The repair process can be so accurate that a radiologist may not be able to detect where the bone was fractured once the healing process is completed. The healing again takes place with the body's own power to do what has to be done.

There are many accounts proving the body's ability to heal itself, but unfortunately, the body can only do so much. In modern society, humans are exposed to many external toxins, which obviously deplete the body's capacity for self-healing. Since it has to struggle against such external forces this healing process can become retarded or stop functioning altogether. As the body keeps getting these toxins dumped into it, it loses its natural healing powers. The body is like a river; while certain pollutants in the river can be tolerated, others need to be extracted by its natural healing forces, such as a fresh source of water from rain...turbulence mixes water with oxygen from various water plants, and the purifier and germicide healers from the sun heals the river. Many plants that grow in rivers, both algae and higher plants, can remove contaminants from water, but the continual dumpling of sludge in water will eventually weakens its natural purification mechanism and as the river becomes overwhelmed, it starts breaking down. As a result, the river becomes sick. This scenario is certainly evident with the human body.

> *"The mine knows naught of the emeralds within its rocks, the sea is ignorant of the gems within its caverns, of its corals, of its sharp reefs, of the tall ships that sail on its bosom, or the bodies that lie buried in the sand, yet these are all there."* -Mary Baker Eddy-

An old story told by Ms. Eddy includes that a man was made to believe that he occupied a bed where a cholera patient had died. Immediately, the symptoms of this disease appeared and the man died. The fact was that he had not caught the cholera by material contact, because no cholera patient had been in the bed. She goes on to say that disease arises like other mental conditions, from association. Since it is a law of mortal mind that certain diseases should be regarded as contagious, this law obtains credit through association, calling up the fear that creates the image of the disease and its consequent manifestation in the body. Therefore, the power within to heal the self may not be obviously visible, but it still remains. All it needs is nurturing, and the right stuff to be put into it.

Since studies show that the mind is responsible for one's health, then truly health can be controlled by thoughts. This gives certain power over one's own health just by thought alone. Individuals who brag about their health and vitality unknowingly are not only planting that concept into their mind but into every molecule in the bodies as well. These types are usually very impatient with doctors (if they ever see one) and have learned to take it upon themselves to learn every facet of self-healing, because of the desire to be in total control over their health. Their cupboards are full of supplements, their refrigerator loaded with fresh fruits and veggies, and they are aware of various natural healing methods, which they keep up regardless if they are sick or not. We can see self-healing can be followed by adherence to a pattern of certain disciplines and also beliefs. In other words, if you think you are well, wish you were well, chances are, you will be well.

BALANCE FOR HEALTH

The Chinese have a saying, "That in all things, one needs to maintain moderation." Their yin and yang symbol indicates two characteristics, aggressiveness (yang) and withdrawal (yin), which humans must strive for to acquire balance and a state of well-being. Today, the word moderation seems archaic in a society distorted by excesses. In a modern society geared towards black and white conclusions with little variable or shades of gray in between, moderation gives overtones of uncertainty and weakness.

Much of alternative healing focuses on both biological and mental balance, which in Oriental philosophy is referred to as yang and yin. Too much yang results in aggressive behavior (stress-related illness), while people with too much yin tend to be submissive and often suffer fatigue. Any form of lifestyle imbalance, such as overindulgence in food, drink, stress, habits, obsessions, etc., results in depleting of other essentials that make up a well-balanced system. Overloading or an inefficient degree of care pertaining to the multitude of human complexities causes imbalance. It is this imbalance which ultimately results in potential illness. As the body requires a large variety of foods to maintain good nutrition, the human psyche also needs a multitude of conditions to keep it healthy.

Individuals who spend hours sitting behind a desk involved in tedious mental work need physical activity to rid the body of inertia. While this balances out physical conditions, the mind also needs to retain balance. The overuse of the left side of the brain, which is involved with tight controlled thinking, needs to be balanced out with the use of right side of the brain, which controls creativity, intuition, and is responsible for tuning up the senses. The latter is achieved through activities that stimulate freedom of creative expression. The use of both sides of the brain maintains balance, thus helping to keep the mind, spirit and body active and healthy.

This sense of balance goes further, and is very subtle but very real. All living things have been endowed with a natural vital source, however, pesticide poisons robs this vitality, thus weakening the plant's natural life source. The well-being of humans can be compared to that of plants. Pesticides deplete the plant's immune system, weakening its resistance to fight off disease as overuse of synthetic medicines, antibiotics, etc., lowers the human's natural immune system. As the plants are weakened, they need to rely more on the vicious cycle of pesticides. With commonsense preventive measures (as with human beings), many of these problems could be avoided. The careful use of organic fertilizers would give plants natural vitality, strengthening their resistance, preventing pest infestation and disease.

DULLING THE SENSES

Our senses have become dulled from overexposure to numerous imbalanced conditions, and are particularly evident in many of our youths' reaction towards life's situations. A sense of numbness and disinterest often is interpreted as "being cool" and has replaced natural curiosity and enthusiasm. Lost to a degree, are feelings of sensitivity and creativity; the subtleties needed to create some form of art have dried up from overexposure to bad entertainment and an imbalanced lifestyle. We need high-powered events to arouse our attention and make us care. We are a nation that overindulges; our energy consumption and waste is the largest in the world. We become frustrated when our unquenchable appetite goes unfulfilled, thus we demand more and more products to maintain a sense of satisfaction. The enormous variety of the most mundane substances, from aspirin items, painkillers, cold remedies, etc., to cereals and cigarettes, available on the market, indicates this excessive behavior. We have fallen prey to commercialism's game of control, the number one rule being the focusing on consumer discontentment. This is achieved through the flooding of a variety of brands of products; the logic being, while what we have may be good, something else must even be better…that commercial said so. Where does this lead us? Any form of overindulgence overturns the scale of balance, the eventual consequences being dysfunction of the mind, spirit or body.

It is more difficult today to find inner peace because of this over- flooding our minds with excessive stimulants, hence places us in the grip of discontentment. Depression and anxiety have become epidemic and threatens those from all walks of life. Perhaps the most vulnerable victims are our youths.

In search for an environment conducive to healing the mind, body and spirit, Gerald Jampolsky, a psychiatrist, developed the first Attitudinal Healing Center in Tiburon, California, in 1975. Using the basic course in "miracles," Jampolsky's original goal was to provide a place where children with life-threatening illnesses could come to take responsibility for their own health. The emphasis was not intended to focus on physical healing but on achieving inner peace. The premise is that any healing process should begin with attitude healing. As the center grew, it started to encompass a variety of programs for people of all ages experiencing conflicts in their lives and seeking counseling for their inflictions. The Person-to-Person Group, the largest group at the center, draws people together to practice positive means of inter-living to share similar concerns and needs. Other concepts, some of which take the form of workshops, are on the topic of the essence of love, being responsible for one's own life, letting go of the past and living for the present, nonjudgmental attitudes towards others, generosity and compassion, seeing life as being eternal, forgiving and forgetting, eliminate the need to command and demand, ridding of the need to feed the ego, yielding towards others, eliminating needs and desires, loving unconditionally, becoming a love finder rather than a fault finder, showing compassion but letting others be responsible for their own lives, and living with peace and tranquility. Perhaps we could add living without the complexities of a multitude of choices to live more simply.

People with terminal illnesses, since they have less to lose, often are more willing to examine such concepts. Since present conditions are so difficult, these individuals often welcome any hint of hope, even if it means accepting something previously not considered when experiencing good health, but sought only after faced with some form of health dysfunction. Under such conditions, alternative healing approaches are more apt to be sought out. Many have waited until all their options with traditional medicine had been exhausted before seeking alternative healing. Unfortunately, this has its shortcomings; it is always better to prevent illness than attempt to cure it after it occurs. Using alternative healing as a means of keeping well, where the immune system is maintained, when illness does strike, tends to be for shorter duration.

CHAPTER 19

HYPNOSIS FOR HEALING

TRICK OR TREATMENT?

Sounds like a medical trick? Yes, surgery without anesthesia is a bit of a mind bender, but the truth is, even in its less startling applications, hypnosis still evokes the image of its sideshow past. Nevertheless, as researchers learn more about the mind-body connection, hypnosis is sneaking, ever so quietly, into various therapeutic fields. Its wide scope of benefits is being recognized in the treatment of life-threatening situations, as well as proving its worth in nurturing processes of self-improvement; to stop smoking, reduce weight, and rid the mind of phobias and depressions. Its added benefits are developing concentration powers, building self-confidence, improving one's skill in many endeavors, and improving feelings of well-being.

Under different labels and since the earliest of times, diverse cultures have practiced hypnosis. The Ebers Papyrus, over 3,000 years old, described the methods used in hypnosis. Egyptian soothsayers' practice of hypnosis is similar to those used today. Tribal shamans, witch doctors and faith healers also used a similar technique for hypnosis but in various different forms. By placing patients in a trance or hypnotic state, the hypnotist enacts certain chants, prayers and symbolic enactments to enhance the desire effects. Except for the lack of props, current techniques are not very different from those of early practitioners. Whether through counting to 100 or asking the patient to concentrate on a peaceful setting, the goal is to relax the body while creating a state of mental awareness that makes it easy to assimilate therapeutic suggestions. An addicted smoker may be told to associate the smell of cigarettes with garbage; a frustrated dieter might be encouraged to crave vegetables.

Helping people kick bad habits is one thing; getting them to take surgical incision without anesthesia is quite another, but Helen Crawford, a psychology professor at Virginia Polytechnic Institute and State University in Blacksburg, says the sensation of pain is like other mental processes that can be controlled to some degree. Her tests of mapping brain waves and measuring cerebral blood flow have shown increased activity in the brain's frontal region, which is known to inhibit sensory information. The pain still registers in other areas of the brain, but the hyped-up frontal cortex blocks its ascent into consciousness.

According to electronic tracings of brain waves from people undergoing hypnosis, there is a surge of theta waves, which are associated with enhanced attention. That may explain why suggestions during this state are so affective. The mind tunes out all sensory perceptions and focuses exclusively on a single thought. The desire for long-term results can also serve as motivation, and experts say that with training and practice almost anyone can use hypnosis for simple healing purposes. In a study sponsored by the government's Office of Alternative Medicine, Crawford taught seventeen people to use this technique to ease backaches; laboratory subjects reduced pain sensation by more than eighty percent. At home, they felt significantly less depressed and were able to sleep better at night. Crawford encourages reluctant individuals by pointing out that self-hypnosis gives more control over their lives. This self-empowerment enables them to self-monitor their reactions to various mental and physical problems they may encounter in their lives. How easily can you be hypnotized? Prior to hypnotic treatment, practitioners will often question their patients to see how they will respond to hypnosis. The following are some of the questions and preparations a hypnotist will ask and follow.

1—Having complete trust in your hypnotist's skills and being willing to follow directions.

2—Capability of concentrating for a period of time.

3—Do you consider yourself to be creative?

4—Do you often rely on your instincts and feelings or methodically use logic to figure things out?

5—Would you consider yourself flexible, willing to take chances or rather be like a creature of habit and need routines?

6—Do you believe there are entities and incidents that may never be completely understood?

7—Would you say you are willing to believe and trust alternative lifestyles, new concepts and ideas?

8—Do you consider yourself adventurous?

If you have answered yes to over five of these questions you are a good candidate for hypnotherapy.

According to New York City psychologist and hypnotic researcher Marcia Greenleaf, hypnotic techniques work by teaching people to use the mind as a "psychological zoom lens." The therapist asks the individual to focus so intensely on a particular theme, thought or idea that external stimuli fade away. A ballerina with a hip pain might concentrate so completely on the music and her steps in the dance that she does not feel any discomfort while performing.

Therapists summon forth the power of suggestion as a way to help patients reduce stress, break self-destructive habits, gain access to unconscious material, and make positive behavioral changes. Greenleaf explains her method: "I ask people to tell me their problems, and then I teach them how to shift gears. First, I show them how to get comfortable. Once in a relax state, I use an ego-strengthening technique to remind them of their attributes and talents."

TESTIMONY

Lanie Torres, a thirty-seven-year-old teacher, mother and artist, consulted Greenleaf because she felt as if her life was spinning out of control. Prior to hypnotizing Torres, Greenleaf discussed the issues that were troubling her. "I'd taken on so many responsibilities at work, with my kids, and volunteering, that one day I just lost it and couldn't seem to get back on track," Torres complained. "Greenleaf put me into a trance, talked about how things deeply known in each of us...that come from love, and told me I could be affirming of myself and still responsible to others. She taught me how to release the notion 'I needed to be perfect' and always serving others while depriving my own needs."

Torres added, "This woman's life changed dramatically in a short time; she quit her job and went back to creating art full-time, cut back on charity work, and stopped being so self-sacrificing with her family."

Hypnosis is not a cure-all for addictive behavior, but it is a popular method of treatment for those who suffer from compulsive overeating. Greenleaf explains, "You can't be completely abstinent from food; rather than simply kicking a habit, you have to learn to control behavior. There are genetic components and emotional issues involved as well." Greenleaf recommends the technique to highly motivated women who are at least midrange in being able to be hypnotized by a therapist and whose problem began in adulthood. A patient who was a good candidate for the "hypnotizing profile" used hypnosis to lose weight, lost one hundred pounds, and has managed to keep the weight off. "After my last pregnancy, I ballooned and tip the scale to two hundred and fifty pounds. Dr. Moshe Torem put me under and gave me the suggestion, *'I could eat whatever I wished but I would have complete control over my body.'* In other words, I would be consciously aware that overeating would have its consequences, and I was responsible for my own condition."

It is amazing how modern doctors and mental therapists are tackling medical problems with an eighteenth-century parlor room entertainment and pushing hypnosis towards the foreground of the medical field. It has become so trusted that surgeons are using hypnosis at the operating table. Supporting hypnosis, many professional physical and mental caretakers emphatically defend this treatment's merits in helping to cure a variety of afflictions…treating addictions, asthma, epilepsy, and hemophilia.

After reviewing medical literature, the National Institutes of Health concluded that hypnosis is effective in easing several kinds of discomforts, including headaches and pain associated with cancer. Mental therapists discovered that hypnosis patients suffering from anxiety, phobias, depression, sexual dysfunction and eating disorders were recovering more rapidly than patients without treatment.

Today, one particular field of hypnosis has proved successful with individuals in the creative arts fields. This kinship evolved because of imagination and fantasy being common roles in each. The capacity for creativity enhances the individual's hypnosis experience. The unwavering concentration during the process of creative acts is similar to the deep focusing that is essential in hypnosis.

Therapists have used hypnosis for releasing creative blocks due to depression. Hypnosis can delve deeply into the patient's subconscious mind so certain problems responsible for inhibiting creativity can be recognized. Some types of creative suppression can be released through encouragement and the long process of psychoanalysis, but patients with deeply rooted emotional problems or even with physical ailments usually are unable to communicate effectively. Hypnosis becomes beneficial when it communicates with the subconscious rather than the conscious mind, thus the hypnotist is able to make positive suggestions to the patient's subconscious mind.

Perhaps the most celebrated use of hypnosis to stimulate creative behavior occurred in Moscow at the turn of the century. Sergei Rachmaninoff for several years suffered deep depression due to the rejection from critics and audience towards his First Symphony. At the time, he became a recluse and claimed he would never again create music. For two years, he had not written any music. Eventually, his depression became deeper, and his friends whom he had not seen for years were afraid he would become suicidal. Finally, they convinced him to see a physician who specialized in hypnosis.

Rachmaninoff was treated daily for thirty minutes over a period of three months. After certain procedures were taken, which are generally used to prepare the patient for the hypnosis process, the hypnotist gave the repeated suggestion to the patient, "You will begin to write again… you will work with great facility…inspiration will flow freely from you… nothing can block it." Rachmaninoff was instructed on how to induce self-hypnosis so he could practice on his own.

Once Rachmaninoff started to respond to treatment, he experienced surges of creative inspiration. In his frequent walks in the countryside, as he looked at nature, music seemed to flow through him. He later remarked that this music that seemed to come from within had to be written down. This period in this composer's life was responsible for his celebrated Second Piano Concerto in C Minor, which was performed in Moscow in 1901 and dedicated to his hypnotist Nikolai Dahl.

Not everyone is a good candidate for hypnosis. Those who are not reluctant to probe in the unknown and have flexibility in thinking and are more receptive to accepting alternative ways of dealing with problems make good patients, whereas pragmatic thinkers, with their black and white method of reasoning, are more difficult to hypnotize. Hypnosis is most effective with patients who believe that it is effective and who have the ability to concentrate deeply, a state in which the mind is most acceptable in receiving hypnotic suggestions.

One major advantage of hypnosis is that it can be self-induced. Self-hypnosis can be more beneficial than a patient-hypnotist relationship because the individual plays a more active part in manifesting the procedure. Being able to conduct techniques, having the potential of controlling major life-threatening diseases, is the ultimate of self- empowerment.

VISUAL HYPNOSIS

Visualization hypnosis is another technique used. Through hypnosis, visions of certain situations, leading to the fulfillment of a desired goal, are the center of focus. It can be visions of acquiring good health and increasing energy; imagery needs to be clear and precise where the individual concentrates on his or her body going through a progressive healing state. With eyes closed and resting in a comfortable position, the hypnotic state can be achieved by visualizing yourself exercising, running, and swimming or engaged any other energetic activity; a peaceful scene works best. Through visualization practice, it is believed such an event can be actualized into reality. Actually, some professional sports individuals claim that prior to their game, they visualized the complete scenario of how they will carry out the various plays of the game. This occurs because while in a hypnotic stage, the subconscious mind has received these images and upon certain suggestions transmits them to the conscious mind, which is used in the daily activity; it's sort of a means of self-motivation.

Past-life regression is becoming a popular parlor room experience. Individuals go into a deep trance, and then they are instructed to go back as far as they can in time, perhaps even centuries; some have experienced digressing as far back as ancient Egypt or biblical times where they took on different roles. Some individuals see themselves as kings, queens, peasants, slaves, and a list of other characters in these past lives. As for health benefits, individuals experiencing a chronic disease can undergo visualization in an attempt to restore their health. Going back in time, when perhaps experiencing good health, the practitioner can make suggestions that the patient feel deeply these past healthy energetic times and have the patient attempt to project them onto the present situation of illness. In a hypnotic state, the patient attempts to regain the past and manifest it into a reality.

Others undergoing hypnosis cannot only envision past events, but futuristic ones as well. One woman undergoing past-life regression envisioned a flood ruining her home. The clarity of her vision included her actually seeing the dirty floodwater entering her beautiful home. A few months later, there was a huge storm and her hypnotic vision was manifested into reality. Another person was able to go back to a place and time in which her parents married. Her vision included a couple wearing traditional wedding attire, the groom in a black suit and a wide-brim hat, and the bride wearing a long peasant-like dress and ribbons flowing from her hair. It was later discovered that her parents were married in Russia and they were wearing traditional wedding clothes.

Self-empowerment through hypnosis, if used correctly, can serve a multitude of purposes. It can alter behavior, open creativity channels, curtail bad habits, excessive drinking, and eating habits, instill self-esteem and courage, and in medical hypnosis, serve as a means of healing. Hypnosis used for healing is effective because patients are convinced, through the subconscious mind, that they are not sick, wherefore we can see how the concept of the mind controlling matter works. That is why hypnosis so often is used for pain control; pain can be often associated with the emotions.

A child running, suddenly falling down, bruising his knee may yell out in pain. The mother picking up the child can charm him from feeling the pain by uttering certain phrases, "You are a brave boy." The child is then encouraged to continue playing and his mind tells him there is no pain. Available on the market are audio tapes which give basic instructions on various methods of self-hypnosis. The process of hypnosis starts with the individual going into a deep relaxed state of mind. By counting from one to ten while mentally visualizing yourself going deeper and deeper down into a void, the individual finally reaches a level of hypnotic sleep. At this stage, the subconscious mind takes over and communicative suggestions are made to correct your illness or addiction; upon wakening, you will retain these suggestions. This awaking process is important because the basic principle of hypnosis is to continue giving guidance to you after the hypnotic state has ended. In other words, suggestions you give yourself while in the hypnotic state will embed in your subconscious and they will be effective in your daily existence.

Now that hypnosis has gained respectability, hypnosis is entering into many facets of life. Those who use its benefits are discovering how it miraculously changes their lives. From parlor room entertainment to the respectable medical field, hypnosis has come full circle, and with the widespread alternative new age movement, it will go even further. So close your eyes and count to ten.

CHAPTER 20

TRIED AND TRUE HEALING METHODS

HOMOEOPATHY

When Elvis Presley died, coroners discovered nine different pharmaceutical drugs in his body. To prevent embarrassment, one of his physicians sought to reassure the public that there were "sound rational medical reasons" for all nine drugs. Such reassurance may have protected Elvis from bad publicity, but ultimately this episode offered a clue to the errors of the medical field in their reasoning that nine pharmaceutical drugs given to a patient at one time could be considered a "sound rational medical reason." What makes this so sad is that this celebrity had access to the best health care, but did not get it. Whatever doctors he used, they were surely highly paid, but their lack of reasoning is frightening in that this could happen in our county's best medical circles and there are many similar incidents which we do not hear about that are occurring all the time.

WORKOUT

Answer the following:

1—How many drugs do you take daily?

2—Are you aware of your drugs' side effects, and if you are aware, what are they?

3—Would you consider making changes in your health care? How far would you be willing to go in your search?

4—Have you attempted to discuss with your doctor if it is possible for you to avoid taking chemical drugs…if there is an alternative route you could pursue?

5—Prior to choosing a physician or health professionals, ask them if they treat patients other than with prescription drugs. Some doctors are integrating natural healing techniques within their practice.

6—Always remember, you choose your doctors, they do not choose you; you have a choice how you are treated. You may be in a position to persuade a doctor to consider an alternative method of healing. As alternative medicine expands, you will find that some practitioners introduce homeopathy in their practice. Make certain you do your homework; check if the homeopathic physician is licensed in your state and belongs to the National Homeopathy Association. You can get this information through the Internet, or have it verified by the practitioner by showing his license and any background information, references and testimonies from other patients.

Actually, you should be going through this process any time you consider alternative healing. While many honorable alternative healers are available, like any other business, there are charlatans who will take advantage of you, so look out for them. Use your local library to do your research on individual healing methods, written by well-known natural healers. You cannot go wrong by reading health advice books concerning alternative healing by Dr. Andrew Weil, a graduate of Harvard Medical School.

Instead of giving patients one medicine for headaches, another for constipation, another for an additional problem, and one to counteract side effects of the given drugs, homeopathy's concept of treating patients is holistic, meaning that one distinctive remedy is given to help build up the patient's overall immune system. Actually, the holistic healer follows this concept throughout your healing process.

BASIC PRINCIPLES OF HOMEOPATHY

The first basic law is patience, because the practitioner needs to sort out cause of illnesses in order to perfect a cure...hopefully, a permanent cure. This is the opposite of traditional medicine, where physicians are more concerned about an instant cure rather than finding the cause of an illness and prescribing a cure.

THE LAW OF SIMILARS

The homeopathic practitioner recognizes that since patients have individual idiosyncratic physical, emotional and mental patterns, even showing up when suffering disease, each patient requires individual treatment. The essence of treatment is that the practitioner attempts to discover exactly what is causing the problem, or the very essence of the cause, and then attempts to find a remedy of that cause without overdosing the patient. Homeopathy defines the underlying principle for this matching process as the "law of similar." Hence, in curing the disease the caregiver gives the patient small doses of a formula until the disease has been eradicated. This concept is known, in traditional medicine, as immunization, which is based on "similars." Except with immunizations, patients are given a heavy dose of the dead disease they suffer from, in which, after the immunization, they are supposed to be immune from catching that disease again. People with cancer are treated with radiation, the element that causes cancer. Digitalis is used for heart conditions, yet digitalis, if used incorrectly, causes heart conditions.

The law of similars is not just a philosophical construct; it is a practical guide to prescribing medicine that heals. Andrea, a fourteen-year old girl, woke up on morning with a sore throat. She complained of swelling and burning pain in her throat. While warm food irritated her throat, cool drink and food helped make it feel better. If one were knowledgeable about homeopathic treatments, they would have been able to detect her symptoms matching up with bee venom. Bee venom causes swelling and burning, symptoms Andrea was suffering from. Bee stings can at times be quite subtle and even overlooked if the sting occurred in midst of an activity. For her healing remedy, Andrea was given a very small homeopathically prepared dose of bee venom, and within less than an hour, she was feeling better. Prepared this way, the drug stimulates the appropriate defense response required for healing.

This method is superior to traditional healing because it encourages the body's own vision to heal itself rather than becoming dependant on some temporary relief, which often works against the body, thus weakening the system.

THE IMPORTANCE OF INDIVIDUALISM

We should avoid comparing our medical problems with others in the attempt to mimic a remedy that perhaps was effective for another individual. Over-the-counter drugs offer temporary relief of the disease symptoms; they are not designed to cure the disease. Holistic healing can be achieved by treating the whole individual, not just focusing on the ailment, but by evaluating the complete person. If you are suffering from a chronic headache, or stomach problems, or depression, you want a permanent healing rather than an over-the-counter drug that makes you feel better for a couple of hours.

In order to find out the true cause of any ailment, the homeopathic physician needs to know exactly what type of complaint you have; a reoccurring headache, a throbbing or dull headache; does it hurt anywhere other than in your head? Does the pain occur behind the head or just in front? Are the headaches accompanied by other feelings of illness; are they worse when you move or when you lie down? What action on your part makes the headache feel better? All these questions are the means the homeopath learns what medicine will best cure the problem (not just temporarily make it feel better).

Sir William Osler, considered to be the father of modern medicine, acknowledged the homeopaths' serious interest in scientific medicine, but there are skeptics who insist homeopathy is not substantiated by the scientific community to be effective. Quite the contrary, there are volumes of studies on homeopathy. We need to go no further in the disputes between conventional medicine and any form of alternate medicine. Nor do we have to indulge into the exact scientific means that make homeopathic medicine so effective. If you wish to become involved in research, there are many books in the market on the subject. This manual is intended to introduce you to the variable natural healing modalities which are becoming part of the of twenty-first century's healing fields.

THE EMPIRICAL EVIDENCE

Whether or not you are convinced, or even interested in homeopathy research, it is worthwhile to look at the following factors:

1—Homeopathy has been practiced on infants and the results are positive. Reports indicate that infants with teething difficulties, feverish conditions, sleepless states, and neurological disorders respond well to homeopathy treatments. Actually, pediatricians should not give drugs to sick children but consider prescribing homeopathic remedies.

(Medical Child Abuse) It is a little-known fact that the vast majority of drugs commonly used for infants' and children's health problems are minimally tested, but still considered completely safe for the age group prescribed. Even a report from the American Academy of Pediatrics admitted that "possibly, as many as three quarters of the drugs used in hospital pediatric practice are not appropriate for use on children" and it is a known fact that pediatricians overdose antibiotics out of fear and expect rapid recoveries. Fortunately, homoeopathy tends to heal more slowly and is more thorough in the healing process. Few parents are aware of the safe effective healing homeopathy provides for their children, nor will their family pediatrician ever inform them. In 1975, the American Academy of Pediatrics recommended that tetracycline not be given to children under eight years old due to liver damage, retardation of bone growth and other problems too numerous to mention. Another study made several years later showed that twenty-seven percent of 1,947 Tennessee physicians were still prescribing tetracycline to children under eight years old, and with the FDA's awareness.

2—The use of homeopathy became very popular in the U.S. and Europe in the 1800s due to its success in treating the epidemics raging during that time; cholera, typhoid, yellow fever and scarlet fever.

3—Homeopathic medicines have the capacity to heal when prescribed in the proper dose. The basic way homeopaths discover what group of symptoms a medicine can treat effectively is through conducting experiments called "proving." This entails giving the patient small doses of a substance once or twice daily for a period of several weeks and then observing the patient for any negative effects or symptoms. The dosage tested is very minute but still measurable. The concentration of the original substance in these doses can be so small that in all probability there are no remaining molecules left of the substance tested. When taking continually, a.c.h. medicine has the capacity to cause its own unique set of symptoms.

PSYCHOTHERAPY: HOMEOPATHIC STYLE

Too often, people assume that psychological problems require psychological solutions. Since some psychological symptoms arise from physiological processes and (vice versa), psychological treatment is of value to treat the patient holistically. A holistic approach is inherent in homeopathic care; a homeopath prescribes to the patient a chosen medicine, but goes even further in giving advice on proper nutrition, provides stress management programs, and emphasizes the relationship between the mind and body in regards to the patient's present health state. Included in this advice is information on environmental determinants of health and disease. The homeopath may also deal with the emotional and mental state the individual is experiencing. Today, some mental therapists, while not having the licenses to issue prescription drugs for depression, will use, in part, some homeopathic techniques to treat the problem.

One particular method used by homeopaths in a psychotherapeutic process for attempting to dislodge a symptom so as to set a curative process in motion is for the therapist to encourage the patient to pretend to experience the problematic emotional state. If a person suffers from a dreadful fear of snakes, he or she is asked to visualize in their mind a huge deadly snake and pretend to be afraid. In this way, the individual understands that his fear is accepted and will not be criticized. This self-acceptance helps to encourage the individual to use his or her inner emotional strength next time they encounter something that is feared. Psychotherapies that recognize the importance of accepting rather than denying one's emotions are a first step toward a "homeopathic" cure.

In a personal situation, I remember when I first started teaching how I feared standing in front of a classroom. I knew I had a fear of public speaking, but somehow it had to be dealt with in order to pursue a teaching career. To cure the problem of "public speaking," I spoke in public until it was cured and eventually became a member of the International Board of Outstanding Speakers. Hence, once I faced up to the reality of this fear, I was able to completely omit it and from then on never feared public speaking. In essence, it was approaching my fear of public speaking by actually doing it that cured me.

This healing method can be seen somewhat in homeopathy where healing is based on likeness heals likeness. That means that whatever the illness, the remedy, in part, comes from the ingredient that causes the illness in the first place. The curing ingredient is diluted to a certain point that makes it beneficial. Included in this method of treatment is the probing into the patient's background and current lifestyle. The practitioner asks many questions, which helps to gain a complete picture of the patient.

ENERGY HEALING

Carol Hannum is an alternative health medical intuitive who performs energy healing through readings and aura cleansings. She bases her healings on those of Dr. Caroline Myss, the guru of intuitive medicine. Ms. Hannum's approach, developed over many years of research, offers a variety of methods to both animals and humans which includes body aura reading, psychic reading, allergy therapy, and cleansing with spiritual cleansing, aura cleansing, and detox of the liver, alcohol and drug detox. The healing comes from her patients believing in miracles and having total faith in her approach.

The beginning of this method deals with the total bioelectrical field in and around the body. She takes a look into her patient's present and past life influences and how they affect their present health, which includes emotional triggers, past emotional and physical wounds the conscious mind has forgotten but the subconscious mind has not. After this emotional body diagnosis and balancing, she then proceeds with what she terms as "sweeping" the organ systems. Using pendulum dowsing and psychic readings with inventory manifests and health index of each part, the healing process begins. With this technique, she is able to acquire pertinent information on what is going on inside the body. This index reading enables her to see the healing process both before and after a patient's therapy of auric clearing or energy healing begins.

Energy Alchemy provides an alternative to using liver cleansers, kidney cleansers, detoxifiers, etc., which she helps her patients do. This unique technique, which is non-invasive to the body, involves a spiritual process, similar to shamanism healing, and just as mysterious. Energy Alchemy is a process which activates a patient's higher self and self-healing energies, it also works with the organs, glands and other internal systems. Vertebrae and discs can be adjusted and restored without the patient going through a traumatic experience...it also aids in the regeneration of tissue and synthesis of nutrients.

Patients with various types of hepatitis have been healed with this technique. Patients have given testimonies after a short treatment period of only twenty-four to seventy-two hours stating that their liver enzymes return to normal, blood tests show no abnormalities, and their urine is no longer dark. Claims have been made that this healing technique also is beneficial for diabetics, enabling them to get off their medication. Clearing or sweeping away toxins in the body helps rid the system of chronic fatigue. While this may sound like a miracle cure, perhaps that is exactly what it is. Research has found that those who believe in miracles are able to be cured by believing they will be cured and have better results than nonbelievers.

With this aspect of healing, which includes psychic tuning, we can start describing what an aura appears to a clairvoyant. The healer being able to see a patient's aura is essential; the aura appears as an egg-shaped swirl encircling the individual. In the average person, this shape is constantly changing in swirling color patterns and is somewhat clear and vibrantly iridescent. The healer studies this aura, its colors and patterns, to detect the patient's mental and physical well-being, as well as such intangibles as the nature of the patient's soul or spirit.

Depending on the individual's level of health, a healthy person's aura will be bright and colorful, on the opposite end, dreary and murky, resulting from some emotional or physical affliction. Along with such intangibles as aura healing, there is energy healing, which deals with the body's own power of self-healing. The high frequency of the hands-on healing called La-Ho-Chi, and practiced by healers who claim this healing method is a profound gift from the universe, uses the "aura touch love method" in their healing practice. It is believed that the physical body is encircled with numerous energy layers, or fields, that vibrate at different frequencies, and any illness or imbalance on the physical/cellular levels also exist as energetic disturbances in the energy field. The higher the frequency of light the healer can access, the more complete the healing will be on every level.

It is said that instruction of how to use this technique was given to a spiritual teacher named Satchamar on May 15, 1991. The "La" refers to the light, love and wisdom coming from the Christ Frequencies. The "Ho" refers to the movement of this energy and the "Chi" is the life force. LaHoChi is healing light of the highest frequencies that moves energy with the combined intentions of spiritual and human beings to wherever it needs to go. It can be used to heal the earth, humans, animals and plants. A unique feature of LaHoChi is that its masters hold in place a "seal of protection" around the healer and recipient, which is believed to guard against vibrational interferences. This protects the healer from negative energies released during healing. It also reweaves the energy field by repairing holes, tears, and shattered areas caused by a variety if impacts from birth, radiation, surgery, drugs, accidents, former and present life injuries, all types of trauma, environmental toxins, negative programs and genetic tendencies.

We are referring to healing processes which utilize the self in unique fashions. We are reminded how fragile but complex the human body and spirit are and that subtleties, no matter how slight, can have either a positive or negative effect. Realizing that our subtle energy bodies play a major role in maintaining our health, we can understand how any energy disturbances in the etheric body precede the manifestation of abnormal patterns of cellular organization and growth. Disease becomes manifest in the physical body only after the disturbance of energy flow has become crystallized in the subtle structural patterns of the higher-frequency bodies. The most effective way to alter dysfunctional patterns in the subtle body is to administer therapeutic doses of frequency-subtle energy in the form of vibrational medicines. To clarify, subtle matter is as real as dense matter; its vibrational rate is simply faster. To alter our bodies, therapeutically, we need to administer energy that vibrates at frequencies beyond the physical plane. What are termed "vibrational medicines" are simply those that contain these high-energy frequency subtle energies. Vibrational medicines are seen in the essences or tincture, which are charged with a certain frequency of subtle energy. A good example of this can be detected in homeopathy remedies. Many vibrational remedies exist from Mother Nature. One in particular can be seen in one of our planet's precious gifts, the flower. Dr. Andrew Weil suggests that keeping fresh cut flowers in the home can be a miraculous healer.

KEY POINTS ON VIBRATIONAL MEDICINE

1—Vibrational medicine's purpose is to balance together the individual with his or her higher self. It utilizes tools that produce energy rather than matter in the healing process. Rather than resorting to materialism healing, patients seek non-tangible means such as prayer, meditation, color and crystal healing.

2—Vibrational medicine exists on the premise that most illnesses are manifested through emotional dysfunction; therefore, any treatments should be based on this theory. Often these emotional problems can derive from such subtleties as changes in life habits…sleep deprivation, diet change, divorce, loss of employments, death of loved one, etc. Vibrational healing develops the individual's inner strength through the use of various healing modalities without the use of any drugs.

3—Since vibrational healing uses more of a holistic approach, which attempts to heal the whole individual, than conventional medicine, its results are slower; it approaches the inner being of the afflicted, and its healing results are more permanent. This healing method is not intended to heal one particular problem but to ensure the sick become more stabilized and balanced so that the immune system can defend itself from the onslaught of any diseases.

BIOFEEDBACK

This practice combines a variety of relaxation methods, such as guided imagery and meditation, with the use of instruments that monitors the individual's response to various situations. After a period of treatments, patients learn to monitor their own various modalities, heart rate, blood pressure, and other processes that are believed to be involuntary. With the conscious effort of regulating these functions through biofeedback, pain and other ailments can be minimized.

During the biofeedback session, electrodes connected to a monitoring unit are taped to the fingers, sometimes on other parts of the body with the patient feeling no pain. The biofeedback machine then measures any number of conditions, including skin temperature, pulse, blood pressure, muscle tension and brain wave activity. As various activities are used, relaxation techniques are employed to lower blood pressure. The machine responds by measuring moment by moment feedback on your progress. The purpose of this is that eventually the patient will be able to reach a state of relaxation without the help of the practitioner or the machine. Some of the best results of this healing technique are helping to cure migraine headaches and just pain in general, and also help patients with high blood pressure.

CHIROPRACTIC TREATMENT

Chiropractic practice is often not accepted in the medical community, mostly because it is a method of treatment that does not use medicine. Although highly trained in their field, chiropractors take a back seat to traditional medical practice. The basic function of chiropractic is to alleviate pain; however, it is used for other purposes through the manipulation of the spinal column. This technique is used on the premise that if the spinal vertebrae are properly aligned, impulses from the brain are able to travel freely through the spinal cord to the various organs, thus maintaining the body's ability to keep working well. The object of chiropractic treatment is to return the spine's alignment to its normal healthy state.

After locating spinal misalignments, chiropractic adjustments are used to get the body back to healthy working order. Adjustments can be made by touching, active motion where the patient bends and stretches in particular positions, applications of heat and cold, electrical stimulation, nutrition and other natural therapies. The essence of this treatment is to get the body in the appropriate condition so that it can heal itself, which falls right into the realm of holistic healing.

THE MACROBIOTIC WAY

It was Hippocrates (460-370), known as the "Father of Medicine," who was the first to use the term macrobiotics. In Greek, *macro* means "large" or "great" and *bios* means life. Macrobiotics means "great life." It was the late eighteenth century when a German physician named Christopher W. Hufeland wrote a book entitled *Macrobiotics*, or the *Art of Prolonging Life*.

The macrobiotic lifestyle, as we know it today, is based on the findings of Sagen Ishizuka, MD, and Yukikazu Sakurazawa. These two Japanese educators cured themselves of serious illnesses with a simple diet of brown rice, miso soup, sea vegetables, special non-traditional teas and other wholesome foods. When Sakurazawa came to Paris in the late 1920s, macrobiotics crept into Western consciousness. Sakurazawa changed his name to George Ohsawa and began teaching the macrobiotics lifestyle. The cornerstone of macrobiotics is a body-friendly diet based primarily on whole grains and vegetables, a diet that takes into consideration the inner workings of the human body.

MASSAGE

Much has been written about this technique, which is growing by leaps and bounds, and one reason is that some insurance companies cover massage therapy under certain conditions, particularly injuries from auto accidents. There is an abundant amount of massage therapists in any city, but caution need be taken in finding one suitable for your needs. Massage falls under the category of bodywork and involves the manipulation of muscles and other soft tissues, and helps with a wide variety of ailments, particularly alleviating pain. By promoting the body to relax, stimulate and increasing lymphatic circulation, promoting blood circulation and help drain sinus fluids are some of the results of this healing technique. Listed below are various massage therapies.

Deep Tissue Massage—This is used to relax chronic muscular tension, deep tissue massage, and is applied with some good deal of pressure to a particular problem area. It is often used in conjunction with chiropractic therapy. This method can be painful, so it is important to choose a professional therapist with the proper credentials, because a poor therapist can do more harm than good.

Esalen Massage—This type of massage attempts to bring about a sense of well-being through deep and beneficial states of consciousness. Esalem massage focuses on both the body and mind as a whole. The massage practitioner massages in a gentle rhythmic fashion that is intended to place the patient in a deep relaxing state. Since it is not a deep massage, it not intended directly for pain relief.

Feldenkrais Method—This method uses two approaches: awareness through movement and Functional Integration. The first technique includes guiding participants through a slow gentle sequence designed to replace old movement patterns with new ones. Functional Integration is an individualized approach that uses hands-on touch and movement. These methods differ from other massages because they do not attempt to alter the body's structure. It is through touch that the practitioner attempts to communicate a sense of improved self-image and movement. **Sports Massage**—This is a combination of kneading the body, stretching and using a range of deep-tissue motions. This massage is designed to ease muscle strain and promote flexibility. It is most effective when applied before and after exercise.

Neuromuscular Massage—This is deep tissue massage, concentrating on a specific muscle, perhaps damaged through injury. By the use of concentrated finger pressure, sensitive "trigger points" are released so that blood flow is increased, which helps to heal the body.

Shiatsu—This literally means "finger pressure" in Japanese. This Oriental technique focuses on acupressure points to restore and maintain health. By applying firm rhythmic pressure on certain areas of the body, the therapist attempts to unblock the energy that flows through the acupuncture points.

Reiki and Shin Do—Both of these are body-mind approaches. The practitioner attempts to put the patient at ease by gently touching or gently massaging the body in various areas while soft healing music is being played. The gentle warm touch acts as a healing, something like a mother's loving touch to the child. The areas focused on are called chakra points in which the practitioner gently touches or lightly rubs in circular motion. People suffering from depression or anxiety can benefit from this therapy; however, it is most important that the patient feels comfortable in the surroundings and with the practitioner, and the environment is loving and caring, which will help to facilitate healing.

PROLOTHERAPY

While there are many promises of pain cures, usually made by chiropractors, acupuncturists, and massage therapists, the following is perhaps the most unique and used by a medical doctor, Donald Carrow, located in St. Petersburg, Florida.

Prolotherapy is a non-surgical natural means to assist the body to repair itself of injured tendons and ligaments. The roots of this therapy dates back to the 1920s and it experienced a resurgence in the 1950s, way before the alternative health movement became active. This technique follows the concept used by Hippocrates, who had a wonderful vision regarding the ability for the body to heal itself. Nature has given us all the necessary ingredients for healing; however, just like nature, things can go amiss, and the consequence is the occurrence of illnesses. To cure this imbalance, the body exhilarates itself for healing. This is where prolotherapy fits in. In ancient times, Greek soldiers with torn or dislocated shoulders endured a hot poker thrust into the joint by Hippocrates, resulting in a miraculous healing of the injury.

An interesting history of prolotherapy includes a patient who, in his forties, was informed of the sad news he would have to expect a lifetime of chronic pain. That patient was a physician who was destined to make his mark as our country's surgeon general, C. Everett Koop, MD. He was so totally committed to this therapy that he offered it to his pediatric patients whenever he observed they were suffering from pain. The physician Dr. Gustav Hemwell, who treated Dr. Koop, was one of the greatest teachers of prolotherapy.

This therapy, an injection technique, using natural substances that cause the proliferation (hence the term "prolo") of new cells where ligaments tissue has weakened. The injection is done in the inflamed area, stimulating the area to draw additional blood flow with nutrients. All this stimulates the tissue to heal itself. This healing cascade results in the body's production of new collagen, which becomes new ligament or tendon tissue. Rarely do damaged ligaments heal back to normal, but studies have revealed this therapy can actually strengthen ligaments that have been damaged. Clinical studies have actually demonstrated increased ligament strength after prolotherapy treatment. Since the substances used for the injection are no longer patentable, there is no financial incentive to promote their use for pharmaceutical drug companies. Instead, what is being produced by the pharmaceutical companies are the prescription anti-inflammatory agents, such as the well-celebrated Celebrex and Vioxx. This is the quick-fix approach, which does not offer permanent healing, but instead camouflages the problem. The European Conference in Rheumatology points out that no prescription drug has ever cured a single case of arthritis.

LIVING FOREVER WITH HBO

Most of us have never heard of HBO (hyperbaric oxygen) therapy and probably could not find a source where we could get treated. Several years ago, federal government agencies decided to disallow cost for unapproved uses of HBO to be permitted as a qualified medical-expense deduction for federal income taxes. California's famous resident and brilliant physicist Dr. Edward Teller, who recently died at the age of ninety-five, icon and founder of the hydrogen bomb and heavy user of HBO therapy, upset with this decision (then well in his eighties), personally testified before Newt Gingrich and also wrote a letter to the president attempting to explain the benefits of HBO therapy. When such a dignitary talks, people listen and the government reversed itself.

Dr. Teller, after enduring a heart attack and several strokes, still enjoyed the mental prowess to be able to continue his work at the Lawrence Livermore Labs across San Francisco Bay, and continued to be a contributing member to world-renowned research teams. His caretaker totally credits his daily home use of HBO in a chamber provided by Dr. Richard Neubauer, who was responsible for the remarkable preservation of Dr. Teller's mind and improvement from his strokes.

COLD LASER THERAPY

We are living in an age where new healing therapies are rapidly entering the medical world. Some are relatively non-traditional and have yet been approved by the FDA, while others, quite unknown, have yet to be approved. As the alternative healing field grows, more healing modalities are being introduced. Oftentimes, a non-traditionalist healer, medical doctors, are responsible for introducing innovative healing techniques. In the medical field, since chiropractors sequestered themselves from the pharmaceutical field, they tend to be more open to these innovative healing fields and willing to put in the time for research and investing in purchasing healing equipment that is usually not available in the general practitioner's office.

Not all the unfamiliar healing modalities being introduced into the alternative healing field are new. Some derived from ancient cultures, acupuncture, massage, yoga, etc. Some have just been invented and entering into the healing field, after going through the FDA approval process of course, are now becoming available to the public. One FDA-approved treatment, which came out in the market a couple of years ago, is the Cold Laser Therapy. It was primarily permitted for use for treating carpal tunnel syndrome, which is a painful debilitating entrapment disorder which interferes with the use of the hands. When left untreated, CTS can cause irreparable nerve damage. Present treatment for CTS consists of anti-inflammatory drugs, rehabilitation through physical therapy, and surgical release of the flexor retinaculum in the most severe cases, all of which have limited success in treatment, thus enabling individuals to return to their normal productive lives.

This is where Cold Laser Therapy plays a strong successful role; this treatment has proven successful in the treatment of arthritis, joint pain, tendinitis, tennis elbow, whiplash, soft tissue damage and neuralgia. This therapy is a non-thermal low-level laser capable of penetrating deep into tissue. In human tissue, the resulting photochemical reaction produces an increase in the cellular metabolic rate, which expedites cell repair and the stimulation of the immune, lymphatic and vascular systems. The result is reduction in pain, inflammation, edema and an overall reduction in healing time.

I personally experienced Cold Laser Therapy from the Rosenthal Chiropractic Clinic in Largo, Florida, and can only conclude here that the lingering shoulder pain I suffered for many years suddenly subsided. Several years ago while visiting some Mexican ruins, I tripped over a rock and dislocated my shoulder. I always referred this incident to a Montezuma curse. Rushed to a shamanistic-type doctor in a small town outside of Mexico City, he yanked and pulled my shoulder attempting to put it in place, but instead fractured it. I was immediately rushed, by emergency jet, to the states and treated by an orthopedic surgeon, and followed by some physical therapy. My shoulder continued to remain stiff and was continually painful. When visiting Dr. Marcy Rosenthal for adjustments, she noticed my stiff shoulder and was surprised it had not healed in all these years. She recommended I take a Cold Laser Treatment, which I had never heard of. Immediately after my treatment, my shoulder felt like I never had the accident.

CHELATION THERAPY

The first thing that comes to mind is, if chelation therapy is so good, why is it not more widely accepted? The following is an excerpt from Dr. James P. Carter, MD, Dr. PhD, who is professor and head of the Nutrition Section, Tulane University School of Public Health and Tropical Medicine, New Orleans, Louisiana.

Most people, including physicians, are not aware or concerned over medical politics, legal machinations and economic sanctions that are controlling factors of the medical practice in the United States. Physicians, or others in the health fields, who may pioneer innovative and nontraditional therapies can be severely criticized from these forces. This is where chelation therapy comes in because it involves a major shift in the scientific paradigm. If such a therapy is accepted this could mean traditional medicine has lost its power and control because it is then questioned as to its validity as being the only means of healing. This in itself can cause an imbalance of politically powerful and well-established branches of the medical profession.

The introduction to such an innovative, non-intrusive, safe

and inexpensive therapy (compared to bypass surgery and balloon angioplasty), which made some surgeons, cardiologists, large teams of health care professionals, and the hospital industry rich and famous in a very quick order.

No doubt, chelation therapy is innovative. Like any new radical therapy when first introduced, it will threaten those unwilling to change their traditional method of healing because they may alter their profession and finances. Such health care people can lose patients, who no longer unquestioningly rely on them for their well-being. Their professional integrity can be jeopardized; the obsolescence of their scientific knowledge questioned, and thus, patients seek other methods of medical treatment. They neglect to understand that if the results of their treatments were successful, patients would not seek treatment elsewhere. Now to explain chelation therapy and discuss what it is all about. It is a treatment by which a small amino acid called ethylene diamine tetra acetic acid (commonly abbreviated EDTA), is administered to a patient intravenously, prescribed by and under the supervision of a licensed physician. The fluid containing EDTA is infused through a small needle placed in the vein of a patient's arm. The EDTA infusion bonds with excess metals in the body and carries them away in the urine. Abnormal metals in the body, such as iron, along with other toxic elements as lead, mercury and aluminum are easily gotten rid of through EDTA chelation therapy. Normally, resent minerals and trace elements, which are essential for health, are more tightly bonded within the body, and can be maintained with a properly balanced nutritional supplement.

Intravenous chelation therapy, with ethylene diamine tetra acetic acid (EDTA), is proven to reverse and slow the progression of atherosclerosis and age-related diseases. Symptoms affecting many different parts of the body often improve. Atherosclerotic blockage to blood flow in the coronary arteries of the heart, to the brain, to the legs and elsewhere is relieved and blood flow increases. The result is that often, bypass surgery and balloon angioplasty can be avoided. Research has recently revealed that even cancer deaths can be reduced by EDTA chelation therapy. The question often comes up, is chelation safe? Many studies have proven that this technique is much safer than heart surgery. Often chelation is questioned for its validity and safety. Just like any other form of treatment, particular attention should focus on the physicians treating the patient, their medical background and their background in the particular field being practiced. If patients agree and feel assured the method being used is the right one for them, then the treatment can be very effective for them. Along with treatment, patients are required to follow a particular lifestyle, such as adhering to a regime of exercise and keeping to a healthy diet. In order for this treatment to be effective, a course of treatments needs to be done, which is the situation with most alternative healing. Since the body is responsible for healing within, it takes time for the healing to take place. If you plan to venture into any type of natural healing, you need patience and faith.

CHAPTER 21

UNUSUAL CURES

GUIDED IMAGERY THERAPY

Dr. Andrew Weil, a well-known nutritional and medical doctor, explained about a situation regarding his wife, Sabrina, who was seven months pregnant and struggling with back pain. Apparently, his wife suffered from a history of back pains associated with childbirth. She usually was able to get relief from chiropractic adjustments but at the time, none was available. There was available another type of help from a friend and colleague of Dr. Weil, Marilyn Ream, a family practice doctor from Washington, who worked in a women's health clinic. Dr. Ream used imagery healing in her practice; she approached Dr. Weil's wife inviting her to participate in her practice, but Sabrina refused because she felt she needed a more mechanical solution.

Marilyn asked Sabrina to lie on the floor, loosen her clothing, and take a series of deep breaths. Interactive guided imagery uses a form of hypnotherapy to induce a state of light trance and communication to the subconscious mind but it goes even further. It inspires the unconscious mind to take on its own role in healing, whereas the patient can connect to it to discover strategies in how to go about healing. The basic purpose is to make the conscious mind aware of this information and act upon it. Actually, in essence, it is a form of self-healing where the patient becomes knowledgeable in how to go about not only healing themselves but also means to prevent such illnesses in the future. This is a practice patients can learn to do on their own whenever they feel a need to heal themselves or are in situations where they feel they may be more vulnerable in acquiring some kind of illness. Most of us are aware that stress is a major culprit in causing illnesses. Recognizing what activities are going to be stressful to the mind and body, the patient can take on this practice when it is most needed.

In this situation, the patient, Sabrina, began her healing process by visualizing herself in a place she felt safe and relaxed. For her, it was a place located in canyon country, Utah. To enhance the reality effect, she focused on smells, sounds and feelings and clearly defined her place of peace. Her facilitator then suggested she shift her focus to her uterus and to the baby inside. Getting in touch with the baby, Sabrina was then told to communicate with her baby and ask it to help make the labor quick and uneventful. She then repeated the words her baby had told her in her reply. Then she was told to return to her peaceful place in Utah. Sabrina was then asked if there were any other issues she wished to cover, to which she replied that she wanted to focus on her back. Mary then told her to put her attention on her back and then Sabrina was to tell her what she saw there. In surprise, she replied that a black area appeared. She then was told to see if this area had anything to tell her. Sabrina said it appeared angry; "It's angry at me," she replied. Her back had responded by telling her to take better care of it and then gave instructions to do so. Following these instructions, Sabrina soon discovered how effective visualization therapy was. Her back was healed and she became a great believer in how such an intangible therapy can sometimes be more effective than hard- core medical treatment. To conclude with this story, Sabrina's baby arrived on time with no negative side results.

INNER VISION AND FAITH (THE POWER OF ONE'S THOUGHTS CAN MOVE MOUNTAINS.)

Various self-imagery exercises have been developed by alternative healing therapists and used for healing. Mental Scientists inform us that the mental pictures we have of ourselves, which alternative practitioners so often refer to as "inner vision," are responsible for human emotion and behavior. Inner vision is responsible for the manner in which we live, and in what we believe. Healing therapists using imagery exercises have their patients see themselves as strong healthy individuals, which are intended to help motivate them into following a healthier lifestyle; this therapy works similar to the "place do syndrome," where healing is based on belief rather than reality. There are testimonials where cancer patients facing near death, and unable to be healed, turned to some sort of faith healing, towards either Christian or various secular faiths. Stunned by this miraculous healing, some cancer specialists concluded these healing were indeed "acts of faith."

THE PHENOMENA OF EFT HEALING

A Personal Testimony

The statement "positive thinking is good for your health" can be equated to "believing can make it so," and holds true meaning in the world of faith healing. Channels and media used for transformational healing—**the sending of healing messages in the form of prayers or dedications to needy individuals,** vary enormously. One only has to experience a Christian church sermon or listen to Christian radio or TV station to understand how a devotee's belief determines the power of a spiritual message and that power can travel beyond the immediate domain of the church congregation. Since the birth of religion from the Christian faith to primitive shamanism, the success of spiritual enactments depended upon the faith of their followers.

One particular form of faith healing, which depends upon the power of faith, is the healing process called "Emotional Freedom," (EFT). While this unusual healing process is not well known, its successes are well documented. EFT is based on patients' faith that this procedure will heal them. The formula is executed in a very structured manner, which requires precise adherence. Like a basic recipe, it has certain ingredients in which the recipe must be precisely followed in order to obtain positive end results. The recipe for this healing method can be memorized, and then each round of it can be performed in about one minute. The full basic recipe consists of four ingredients…two are identical. They are:

1—The Setup
2—The Sequence
3—The Gamut Procedure
4—The Sequence

The following offers a brief description:

The body's energy system is subject to a form of electrical interferences, which can block the balancing effect of this procedure. This potential blockage must be removed or the basic recipe will fail. In other words, in the *setup* stage, you need to make certain your energy system is properly oriented before attempting to remove its disruptions; emotional negativities interrupt any healing process, and need to be gotten rid of in order for healing to become manifested. That explains why some individuals suffering from chronic illnesses cannot be effectively treated. They are unable to turn off some negativity that has plagued them, thus causing their illness. It is like putting the batteries in a tape recorder wrong. The polarity reversal has an official name, "Psychological Reversal," and represents a fascinating discovery with wide-ranging applications in…*all areas of healing and personal performance.* It is caused by self-defeating negative thinking, which often occurs subconsciously and outside one's awareness; to add this self-sabotage hinders the EFT healing process. That is why some of this technique fails; it is up to the technician to help the individual get rid of it through discussion and only then can this healing procedure continue.

The setup works like this; repeating an affirmation three times while rubbing particular sore spots. There are two sore spots; they are located in the upper left and right portions of the chest and you find them as follows: Go to the base of the throat and poke around this area. There is a U-shaped notch at the top the sternum (breastbone); from the top of that notch go down three inches toward the navel and over three inches to the left or right portion of the chest. This is where the sore spot is located; vigorously rub the spot while repeating the affirmation as mentioned above. This action appears strange, but for some reason it is the beginning of the setup. The affirmation goes like this: Even though I have this, I deeply and completely accept myself.

The blank is filled in with a description of the problem the individual is experiencing. Example: Even though I have this *depression*, I deeply and completely accept myself.

The list is long because EFT can be helpful for physical, mental, and emotional ailments.

Next is the sequence, which is a very simple concept. It involves tapping the end of the fingers on the end points of the major energy meridians in the body and is the method by which the "zzzzzt" in the energy system is balanced. The tapping of the tips of the fingers includes tapping with the index finger and middle finger. The tapping is done firmly about seven times on each point while repeating the reminder phrase. The meridian points are at the beginning of the eyebrows, just above and to the side of the nose and on the bone bordering the outside corner of the eye. Tap on the bone under the eye, then just under the nose and midway between the bottom lip and end of the chin. Tap the sternum at the side of the bottom just under the armpits. The inner side of each fingertip is tapped with the two fingers and the middle on the outside of the hand.

The next step is called the Nine Gamut Procedure, which is perhaps the most bizarre-looking process with EFT. Its purpose is to fine-tune through the process of certain eye movements. The eyes are shut tight, quickly opened, and again repeated. A circle is drawn in the air by the healer with the intention of the patient following it with his or her eyes. This is repeated and followed by the individual humming a nursery rhyme for two seconds, and then rapidly counting up to five.

Perhaps for some readers, this assortment of details is confusing, but my personal success from this treatment, which was close to phenomenal, inspired me to tell it all. My initial encounter with this unique healing treatment was by reading a health newsletter on pain and acupuncture and EFT. The information regarding how chronic pain and other ailments could be successfully treated by the releasing of negative emotional patterns that many of us collect throughout the years, sparked my personal experienced research...I took the plunge.

Entering this clinic was a lovely experience in itself and far removed from the usual cold sterile clinical appearance. Beautifully decorated with an oriental flair, with sweet oriental herbal aroma perfuming the air, I was greeted by a charming Chinese healer, Eva Chang, the owner of Pathways to Health in Clearwater, Florida. It was not until I was led to one of the treatment rooms did I realize I was not in "la-la" land but there to get treatment. Ms. Chang, a Chinese physician and primary acupuncturist, gave me a treatment with the needles. Then, peering at me in a quizzical manner as though studying and wondering about me, she startled me by saying, "I would like to introduce you to a special kind of treatment; you may feel it to be bizarre." She added, "Its success depends upon your willingness to believe it will heal you." Needless to say, I was a bit apprehensive, but she reassured me of its validity. Ms. Chang felt I would be a particularly good candidate to be introduced to such an unorthodox treatment. I felt specially honored when she exclaimed that only a select few were offered this treatment, those she felt would understand and accept it. Still my apprehension remained; was I being used as a guinea pig? Would this stuff really work?

In anticipation and profuse perspiration, I propped myself up on the treatment table and waited for the beginning of this mysterious procedure. Ms. Chang then began the treatment. When completed, she offered instructions on how I could follow this procedure on my own. She reminded me that persistence, having faith, and following the exact pattern of the treatment would have positive results.

After many years suffering with dermatitis and seeking help from allergists, dermatologists, medical doctors, and several alternative-type remedies, I finally was able to find relief through EFT.

I need to add that being able to "talk it out" and discuss what I felt was the underlying emotional causes that initially triggered my affliction was a vital part of this treatment. At this time I will not go into detail of what I felt were past emotional problems that were involved; however, I will emphasize that with "talk therapy," I was able to summarize how my negative emotions were causing my physical problems. Can you imagine, even chronic dermatitis can result from one's level of emotional well- being?

"While there are many things invisible to the naked eye, we still believe in them; if we were to only believe what our eyes could see our world would be very small."

WORKOUT

(The following are reminder steps to take in EFT treatment.)

1—You need to be open-minded and willing to look into various healing modalities regardless of how unfamiliar or strange they appear to you. Much of our illnesses occur beyond our scope of understanding; methods used in alternative healing may appear provocative and difficult to understand. Be willing to learn new approaches to healing…do not discount that which appears strange.

2—Make certain you find a reputable healer, particularly in healing fields that are unfamiliar to you. Do your homework; there is plenty information out there for the asking and taking.

3—Once you found a good healer make certain you follow his or her instructions. If you have questions about the treatment, do not hesitate to ask.

4—Avoid discussing your unorthodox healing treatments with your family doctor, even friends and family, unless you believe they will be sympathetic and understanding. You will find that some will attempt to discourage you and perhaps even ridicule your innovative pathway to health.

I always tend to feel a bit hesitant when discussing my personal successful healing experiences for fear that what worked for me may not work for others. However, a treatment as profoundly beneficial as EFT, I felt I had to share. After a year, since my last treatment, my allergy problem still does not bother me. With great diligence, before bedtime, I go through the exact process I was instructed when I was under the care of my wonderful oriental shaman, Eva Chang. In a way, this chapter is dedicated to her and I would like to believe there would always be a place for me on her healing table. In conclusion, if I should ever suffer from any form of illness, I will without hesitation seek out the phenomenal healing of EFT.

FLOWER HEALING

Dr. Edward Bach of England is the most respected in this form of healing. As a well-renowned homeopathic doctor in London in the early part of the twentieth century, he became famous for his Bach Flower remedies practiced in many parts of the world. The process in which he introduced "Flower Healing" was his method of retrieving the essence of flowers for healing many diverse ailments. Similar to homeopathic medicine, flower essences contain minute quantities of physical substances, but still they are considered to be in the category of what is referred to as "vibrational healing."

Dr. Bach was a pioneer medical thinker who was one of the first healers to connect human emotions, such as stress, anxiety and depression as often being the cause of physical ailments. Prior to his alternative healing practices, Dr. Bach was an orthodox physician specializing in bacteriology at a major hospital in London. He was known for his early discovery in his field which related to the presence of particular bacteria found in the gastrointestinal tract of persons suffering from various chronic ailments. He discovered that a number of bacteria which were present in the gastrointestinal tract could be associated with persistent exacerbations of chronic illness such as arthritis and rheumatic disorders. His research included the developing of certain vaccines made from these intestinal bacteria, which would act as cleansers of these bacterial poisons. Based on this assumption, he concocted diluted vaccines from the suspected intestinal pathogens, which he believed were responsible for contributing to certain chronic physical disorders.

In time, Dr. Bach, as a psychic "sensitive," started to observe the effects of flower healing. Living in the hectic lifestyle of London, he had become very ill, which nearly took his life. He decided to turn to nature, which included his long walks in the countryside. His sensitive nature enabled him to touch the morning dew on a flower and feel its therapeutic healing energies. His process of determining all thirty-eight flowers used for remedies was such an emotional and physical strain on him that he died at the relatively young age of fifty-six.

Dr. Bach's process of extracting the healing essences from flowers was gathering the morning dew from flowers bathed in sunlight and dewdrops from the shaded flowers. He then examined them to compare their level of energy and discovered sunlit flowers were higher in this vibrational energy. He was able to place flowers in a bowl of water then placing them in the sun was able to render powerful healing tinctures.

In 1979, Richard Kaatz established the Flower Essence Society (FES). This establishment provided a framework for those working in this healing field to exchange their discoveries. One particular finding was that flower healing worked particularly well with emotionally disturbed and depressed individuals. Certain individual flower essences had the power to relieve such issues as fear, sexual limitations, and helped to manifest psychic and spiritual development. The question arises as to how the mechanisms by which the energies of the flowers are transferred from the water to the human system are answered in the following. Flowers are the highest concentration of the life force in a plant, and act as the fertility process of the plant. They are the combination of the etheric properties of the plant and are at the height of the life force. Essences prepared from the flowers are dealing with ethereal vibration of the plant; the intelligence of the flower is derived from the sun's process of osmosis, and then transferred to people when they assimilate these vibrational energies.

When a flower essence, a homeopathic remedy, is ingested, it follows a specific path through physical and subtle bodies and is assimilated into the circulatory system. Next, the remedy settles between the circulatory and nervous systems, then to the meridians, which Oriental medicine refers to as energy points of the body. From the meridians, the energies reach the chakras and the various subtle bodies. The life force of the essences and remedies seems to be amplified and processed at relay points such as the chakras to enable the energies to be properly utilized by the cellular systems of the physical body. We could go more in detail with this intriguing healing process but that may take another chapter.

In the meantime, there are books on Bach's flower healing available for further study.

MAGNETS

There has been much discussion of the pros and cons of magnets as being useful in healing. Carlos Valbona, MD, a rehabilitation medicine specialist at the Baylor College of Medicine, has scoffed at the idea of applying magnets to the skin to relieve pain. His curiosity was aroused when more and more patients were informing him of their positive experiences with magnet treatment, like how it worked on their particular pain. He started to look into the treatment and ignored the negative comments made, such as, "Magnet treatments as being quackery made by those outside the field of alternative medicine."

His first patient was a priest with post-polio back pain so severe that he could not lift his hand to bless his parishioners. He told the priest about magnet therapy and warned him that he had never tried it and it was not approved by the FDA. The desperate priest agreed to try the treatment so Dr. Valbona placed just one magnet on the priest's back and instantly he felt relief from his back pain. The priest came out of the examination room exclaiming, "It's a miracle. I can raise my arm." Encouraged by this result, Dr. Valbona decided to make his own study on the effect of magnet healing even though his colleagues argued against it. He offered the magnets to fifty subjects, half of whom would receive a placebo for their pain, a dummy magnet, and the others… magnet therapy.

The results were outstanding. Seventy-six percent of the magnet-treated patients reported pain relief during a forty-five-minute treatment, compared to only nineteen percent of the placebo patients. These findings, in a double-blind study, are impressive. While there are still skeptics, Americans spent an estimated $200 million on magnets in one year. No one really knows how this treatment works and why it is so beneficial to some patients. It is believed, by some experts, that magnetic energy alters the chemical interactions in nerve fibers that are responsible for pain impulses. Other thoughts are, "the effect is due to increased blood flow to the affected area."

It is becoming more difficult for doubters when studies keep proving the effectiveness of magnet treatments. Another study was taken by the Richardson Orthopedic Surgery located in Texas. The researchers studied sixty-one patients who underwent disc surgery. Some patients received surgery alone, the rest received surgery followed by pulsed magnetic treatments. The amazing result was that patients receiving magnetic treatment experience a success rate almost twice that of patients receiving surgery without this therapy. X-rays and interviews were used so researchers could use both objective and subjective analysis to determine the benefits of the magnetic healing. While magnets are certainly not a cure-all, they do play a role in alternative healing and unlike pharmaceutical drugs, do not have harmful side effects.

COLOR THERAPY

This perhaps, of all alternative treatments, is the most questionable for many, particularly the conventional medical field where there is little consideration for healing other than from rigid scientific methods. Color therapy is simple and pleasant, perhaps too simple for some to accept as a valid healing approach. Dr. Robert Jay Rowen claimed that one of his patients complained of a swollen goiter and blood tests confirmed her thyroid was inflamed. Nothing seem to cure her, and after attempting hormones, supplements, and even various natural healing remedies, all was to no avail. The doctor then remembered a remedy his nurse had informed him about earlier. Being a scientific healer, which medical doctors are, he was suspicious about the remedy she brought up, which was color therapy. Wishing to help his patient, and with means that were non-invasive, he decided to try it, knowing that no harm could result from the attempt. For the first treatment, Dr. Rowen treated his patient's thyroid area for sixty minutes by flooding the area with blue light. The patient took this treatment for a month on a daily basis and Dr. Rowen reported that the result was miraculous. The therapy, as simple as it was, consisting of just shining a blue light directly on the affected area, cured the patient.

Dr. Rowen explained that color therapy is not as odd as it first appears. He had observed, in his early practice, how a patient suffering from pain and swelling showed huge improvement from using laser stimulators on specific acupuncture points. One patient was instantly cured of debilitating upper back pain from just one treatment. The doctor explained how he had been a longtime believer in the healing effects of infrared light, which included a penetrating frequency delivering heat deep inside the body, thus improving circulation and ridding the body of toxins.

It is difficult to believe color can be so powerful. Perhaps looking back in high school science, you can remember studying how different lights have varied wavelengths; violet has a short wavelength while red a much longer one. The longer the wavelength, the slower it vibrates. Our bodies consist of tiny electromagnetic particles that also vibrate. When the body is stroked with color and light, the latter influences vibration of those electromagnetic particles and in turn, affects the way the body functions; various bands of the light spectrum result in diverse effects in the human body. Projecting a part of the spectrum, such as blue, onto a distressed body area causes the healing effect to occur instantly. For the healing of asthma attacks, purple helps give relief, while indigo is used for healing burns and relieving pain; lemon and magenta are beneficial for numerous other problems, and orange helps with digestive problems. Every color helps with an individual disorder. It is difficult to believe that such a simple therapy can be so effective. Much research has gone into color therapy and those who are innovative enough to try such a therapy have discovered its great benefits. Dr. Rowen believes so much in this therapy that he is making a free offering to send his readers eleven color filters and written instructions on how to use them. His contact number is 800-728-2288.

Frequency energy, also referred to as vibrational healing, such as color therapy, can be explained as follows: If you have ever seen old films where an opera singer, singing a high note, shatters a crystal glass without physically touching it, then it is easier to understand the impact a frequency can have on an object. All matter oscillates or vibrates; this is evident in how frequency hits our ears and vibrates the eardrum to produce sound. Frequency can hit all parts of the body, creating oscillation, which can induce physical effects, both positive and negative. A free thinker, not bound by dogmatic conventions, Dinshah Ghadiali, born in 1873 in Bombay, India, wrote that color therapy was a major source of inspiration and teaching on this healing practice. Receiving electrical training and a medical education, he was not held back by these formal trainings and even was a member of the controversial spiritual Theosophical Society. One of his society colleagues had developed a severe case of mucous colitis and did not respond to any conventional medicine available at that time. Dinshah was convinced the only way his friend could recover was the use of unconventional healing techniques. Recently reading a book on the discussion of the healing practice of chromo therapy, he proceeded with a technique described by Dr. Edwin Babbitt in the *Principles of Light and Color* (1878). Lacking modern conveniences, he resorted to the use of a simple method of shining the light of a kerosene lantern through an indigo-colored glass bottle onto the dying woman, and eventually, after a series of treatments, she was able to rise out of bed.

Another remarkable recovery was experienced by an eight-year-old child. Published in the *Atlanta Medical Journal* in April 1927 by senior surgeon Kate Baldwin, then thirty-seven years into practice, the article described her use of color therapy on the patient. The child was suffering from extensive and severe burns; a high fever of 105 to 106 degrees and most shocking, there was no urine output for more than two days. Despite forced fluids, the child failed to urinate. To make matters worse, fluid loss from burns can deprive the body of essential fluids and with not enough blood to pump through the kidneys can lead to renal shutdown; this is a feared complication of burn and crushed injuries. There were other complications that Dr. Baldwin had to face, and against all odds, she did not give up hope. Her treatment consisted of applying the color scarlet over the kidney areas at a distance of eighteen inches for twenty minutes. Alarmingly, after two hours, the child voided eight ounces of urine.

Dr. Baldwin stated the following, "In thirty-seven years of active hospital and private practice, in medicine and surgery, I can produce quicker and more accurate results with color than any or all other methods combined, and with less strain on the patient. Color is the simplest and most accurate therapeutic measure yet developed."

There is much evidence that the sun heals. Although it has gotten a bad reputation due to its cancer-causing properties, still the benefits outweigh the negatives, which by the way, is always given as an alarm signal by deadly white-skinned dermatologist. True, too much sun has a nasty result of causing wrinkles, but other than that, nothing is healthier then bathing in direct sunlight; half-hour dose, daily. This is about the same amount of time color therapy is used on patients. While we are on the subject of color therapy, the question rises, why doesn't the sun heal every ailment since all the colors are contained in sunlight? While the sun has all the colors of the rainbow, the therapeutic effect of one frequency can be unbalanced or neutralized by the presence of another frequency.

MORE WAYS TO USE COLOR

Art therapy utilizes the concept of color as a means of diagnosing the mental well-being of patients; bright colors, such as oranges, pinks, yellows, greens, and sometimes red, give an indication that a patient's state of well-being is fairly good. A patient's fixation on the use of the primary color red can represent states of anger or immaturity. Whereas, if a patient's constant choice in their art works are blacks, grays or dark blues this is an indication these patients are suffering a degree of depression. Actually, art therapy can be a means of approaching patients with certain mental disorders. By encouraging patients to visualize brighter colors for their art work and then to use them as they see them internally has in some situations helped patients to raise their sense of well-being. Severe mentally handicapped individuals who have been immersed in art therapy for a period of time, with the assistance of a competent therapist, have been known to improve their quality of life. As the patient's mental state becomes well adjusted through art therapy, their choice of color in their art brightens and their condition becomes more defined. It is as though they are expressing their ability to better discern reality from their past unreal world. A well-known healer, Rudolph Steiner, used mental color imaging for healing his patients. He would instruct his patients to meditate and visualize a particular color bathing the afflicted body area. Holding that image, the color was believed to wash away the affliction, as if the color was some kind of healing water.

FOOD AND COLOR

There are yet more ways of getting color into the body. Science has proven that colored foods are better for us then colorless foods because they contain beneficial pigments of the bioflavonoid family. The color of food may have influence in energizing or activating molecules; foods do fit the color spectrum.

Red foods include radishes, beetroots and red fruits, such as cherries, strawberries and raspberries and certain plums.

Orange foods include yams, oranges, squashes, apricots, persimmons, cantaloupes, peaches and carrots.

Yellow foods include pineapple, yellow corn, lemons, yellow squashes, and yellow peppers.

Blue foods are rarer but there are blueberries and blackberries; these foods have great detoxing assets.

Violet foods include eggplant, purple grapes, certain berries, purple broccoli and purple asparagus.

Basically, foods that are dull in color or just colorless, such as most sauces and gravies, meats, potatoes, and pastas are not as nutritional as bright-colored foods.

GUIDED IMAGERY

Much research has indicated that bodily functions previously considered to be beyond conscious control can be modified using psychological techniques. Guided imagery, a growing popular healing practice, uses the mind's body connection to help patients rid themselves of pain. It is believed that one can actually think away pain by positive thinking. A successful person, busy with a world of activities, tends to feel pain less than one who is suffering from mental anxieties and depression. Current research has established a link between negative emotions and the lowering of the immune system; they concluded that positive emotions build up the immune system.

Guided imagery, a healing method, functions as a means of the mind seeing certain mental pictures of situations in pictures. This visual process can help build up positive thinking by visualizing certain positive images. In guided imagery, the mind conjures up certain mental pictures or scenes in order to direct the body's energy. If you have cut your finger, you can visualize the immune system starting to work healing the wound. You can actually visualize the cut stop bleeding, closing up and getting better. People with cancer have been known to heal through intense imagery practice by seeing cancer cells actually melting away. In other instances, rather than focusing on pain, individuals can visualize positive pictures, such as it being a beautiful day with lovely landscapes and ocean scenery. This technique is also used for healing rheumatoid arthritis, reduces high blood pressure by lowering stress. Taught properly, guided imagery can be an effective form of self-care. While your doctor needs to be part of your healing, you can add this powerful healing method to speed up the

healing process.

Most of these treatments I have personally experienced, and had the opportunity to discuss them with various practitioners. All attempts were made to contact the very best in each field so as to pass pertinent information to my readers. While these treatments are considered unusual, although effective, they are unavailable in traditional doctors' offices. Through research, you can find them, some of which may be located within your area. Make certain that whomever you choose, you do your homework and check on their background. Listed throughout this manual are means and ways to go about doing this.

CHAPTER 22

TAKING SUPPLEMENTS

SUPPLEMENTING A POOR DIET

Since the average American modern diet is so lacking, many alternative health physicians suggest taking supplements to make up for nutritional deficiency. This includes taking a quality multivitamin, available only in health stores or through an alternative healer. It should provide at least 500 mg of vitamin C and 50 to 75 mg of all of the B vitamins, 10,000 units of beta-carotene and 5,000 to 10,000 units of vitamin A. It should also include 200 mcg selenium and 15 to 30 mg zinc. If a multivitamin does not provide these nutrients, taking a teaspoon of cod liver oil daily and also adding an extra gram or two of vitamin C, to help avoid infection, is recommended. If flu is coming on, 3,000 mg more of vitamin C is recommended for several days. Following such a regimen helps relieve dependence on prescription drugs, because the overall immune system is strengthened against the onslaught of diseases.

While supplement companies abound, and more are sprouting out daily, certain precautions need to be followed; doing research on these companies pays off. Supplements should never be purchased in drugstores or general food markets, although this is perhaps the most convenient means of acquiring them. Usually inferior, these vitamins contain fillers and are not properly processed; using the dry-freeze method hinders the nutrients in the supplements. Instead, supplements should come from a reputable health food store or health practitioners.

One way to do research is through the Internet where well-known brands of supplements can be pulled up and researched to determine the purest quality. Several books are available from reliable sources on the subject to help with this screening. There are also numerous books with hyped claims of remedies that are a cure-all or offer to heal chronic ailments overnight; stay away from these books...they are dangerous. Such unsubstantiated claims are intended to persuade those who are desperately seeking a cure to purchase their product and their information is dangerous and unreliable.

MAKING THE BEST CHOICE

The basic difference between pharmaceutical drugs and natural healing remedies is the former offers immediate relief for physical ailments but rarely offers permanent healing, just temporarily covers the symptom. On the other hand, natural methods, while requiring more time to work than prescription drugs, gradually heal the body because they works with the body's own energies, thus, healing is more permanent. Obviously, during suffering, the remedies promising immediate relief are preferred, which for some, justifies the use of pharmaceutical drugs. One solution: Along with taking a prescription drug, an appropriate supplement is taken which enhances the healing process, and then gradually the drug is weaned off. When an antibiotic is prescribed, an herbalist will recommend taking certain herbal remedies to put back the good bacteria in the body that the antibiotic destroyed. *Lactobacillus acidophilus* is a good source for replenishing bacteria destroyed by antibiotics. For severe flu conditions, or chronic infectious sinus, when a prescription is prescribed, alternative healing remedies include the taking of echinacea and goldenseal, which are excellent remedies.

The Food and Drug Administration does not accept the validity of herbs and vitamins as cures and actually in the past has issued warnings against them. It is true that some contaminated herbs have come from China, but such situations are rare and can be avoided. With certain precautions from the FDA more control over such contaminated herbs getting into the country are being made but the FDA is limited to what it is willing, or perhaps capable of doing in controlling every supplement and herb; individuals are on their own.

This sort of responsibility requires making good substantial choices and having the patience and discipline to search out quality products to ensure they maintain the highest quality available. After all, your health, your very life, depends on how you go about seeking such means in approaching your problems. With the growing emergence of information, scores of miraculous testimonies on personal successful healing using variable natural means, many have indeed, been able to make excellent choices in their health maintenance and also have made miraculous recoveries from lifetime illnesses.

Replacing medical drugs, from traditional medical care, with supplements and natural healing to allow your body to heal itself in a natural way, requires dedication and work, but there are professionals in the field who can be of great assistance. Dr. Robert Jay Rowens from Johns Hopkins University has a newsletter called "Second Opinion," which is packed with useful information on alternative practitioners and supplements. Dr. Andrew Weil, a graduate of Harvard University, has written several books on natural healing, one called *Spontaneous Healing*. Dr. David Williams, who travels the world in search for the most recent finds in herbal healing supplements, particularly Australia, where he is in touch with local customs and their herbal healing methods, offers excellent advice on herbal healing.

PROS AND CONS OF SUPPLEMENTS

Taking supplements is best taken under a specialist's care, either an alternative practitioner or a competent nutritionist. As for quality, the finest source of supplement distributors can be found through *Prescription for Nutritional Healing*, written by James F. Balch, MD, and Phyllis A. Balch, CNC. This thick-volume health encyclopedia, updated yearly, can be found virtually in every health food establishment and in many alternative healing clinics where health specialists use it as a research guide.

Also listed in this book are specialists and instructions involved in various healing fields, which without this source of information, they would be almost impossible to find. Listed is this volume are the phone numbers for hotlines: AIDS, Alcohol and Drug Helpline, Meat and Poultry hotline, Lung Disease, Child Abuse, Poison Control, etc. Listed in the back of this manual are some useful contact numbers and various supplement companies that are reputable and trustworthy for the quality of herbals and supplements they sell.

A CLOSER LOOK

Many so-called natural healers using an assortment of healing methods have sprung up in the past decade. Being aware of the desperate state some individuals find themselves in seeking relief from their family physicians leaves doors wide open for potential charlatans. Any health practitioner promising miracle cures for every ailment needs to be scrutinized as to their validity. Obviously, this includes taking a closer look into any type of claim made regarding some form of overnight miraculous healing. The herb Ephedra, which has just been pulled off the market due to some related deaths, has for years made promises of weight loss. Overweight desperate people gobbled it up like candy, knowing of its horrendous side effects...interaction with anti-depressants and blood- pressure medication, causing high blood pressure or an increased heart rate. Herbal companies that manufactured Ephedra are up in arms and still making claims of its positive usage.

Congressional investigators recently dealt a blow to the Food and Drug Administration's planned crackdown on ephedrine-laced dietary supplements. To justify their actions, they accused the agency of sloppy science. In 1997, the FDA proposed mandating warning labels and a dramatic slashing of the dose of ephedrine in herbal supplements, citing of 17 deaths and 800 illnesses linked to products promising weight loss, building muscle and heightening sexual performance; the FDA created a storm of protests and accusations from the users of the supplement. The Congress General Accounting Office doing the investigation agreed it was justified in investigating this drug. It was concluded that health officials were negligent in their conclusion that supplements should contain no more the eight milligrams of ephedrine per dose. Studies suggest twenty milligrams may be the dose at which certain individuals suffer side effects. However, the FDA, with inaccurate research, focused on thirteen reports of severe illnesses; from this proposal, they determined that a much lower dose would have to exist before this substance would be safe for human consumption. Some agree that this decision is inexcusable for such a vital health hierarchy. Some also believe the FDA's decisions on health issues to be gospel. The FDA acts as one of the most important regulatory agencies in government. For the FDA to use the adage "poor science" to reprimand a health product or health product manufacturer is inexcusable since they omit such language when referring to a chemical medical manufacturer. Hence, this raises warning flags for other products this agency regulates in its prejudice against health supplements and health supplement manufacturers.

The American public is inundated with commercials pertaining to super cures, coming from all directions; TV, radio, newspapers, and health newsletters, which are becoming more predominant then ever. Some of these health fixes appear super miraculous, promising overnight cures for those suffering from seemingly incurable chronic diseases. When an individual suffers a long-term affliction, no matter how ridiculous some of these cures appear, they tend to grab onto whatever is out there…a hurting person is vulnerable. What makes matters worse is if this particular cure does not work, he or she is more than willing to continue their search for the magic fix. This is exactly the reason why some individuals have turned their backs on natural healing. Just a small dose of negativity publicized in the news and you face "I told you so!" attitudes. There are many just waiting for a reason to turn their backs against natural healing and use the overly repeated confirmation, "It has not been accepted by the FDA." Not too long ago, research came out announcing that the herb echinacea was damaging to the liver. Nothing was said that if used on a long-term basis this damage could possibility occur and only with those with weak livers. The word got around that echinacea is bad for you because it destroys your liver. Individuals fail to realize that like any drug, supplements need taken as prescribed, and any overdose will have negative consequences. Much of the public, when it comes to their health, does not think for themselves and depends solely on the discretion of their doctors. We are willing to acknowledge and use our freedom of speech, the right to vote, to make critical choices in our lives, but when it comes to our health, our self-determination flounders. We become intimidated and powerless and neglect to realize, even in our health, we can have the power to choose how we go about healing ourselves.

There are many pros and cons in the field of natural healing, just as there is in life. Differentiation needs to be made between what is good in natural healing and what is not. The big craze regarding calcium supplements to prevent osteoporosis, so readily seen on TV commercials, has raised some skepticism. Dr. Constance Kies of the University of Nebraska remarked, "Taking calcium supplements may actually make osteoporosis even worse." Diets are seldom deficient in calcium, although absorption of calcium may be a problem. It is more likely that deficiencies are in magnesium, manganese and vitamin D, which helps bones to absorb magnesium. Too much calcium consumption can result in calcium buildup around joints and soft tissue…results…the consumer believes the calcium buildup or lump is cancerous…resulting in a painful and dangerous biopsy to determine its origin.

Another supplement publicized to be a cure-all and toted by some hobbyist alternative healers is colloidal silver. People hear that this supplement is a wonderful natural antibiotic that kills germs, disease, virus and fungus and rush to acquire this wonderful healing miracle. Only part of this is true. Most colloidal silver is only safe if taken externally and if taken by mouth can be toxic. Silver if absorbed through the intestinal tract can produce negative results, as with any heavy metal. In colloidal silver, it is difficult to control the concentration of the silver and more importantly the particular size.

There is a product considered safe for sore throats and nasal infection, which is distributed by a company called DEDI and available at heath supplement stores. Colloidal silver does have a valid place in medicine but it needs to be used with caution and certainly is not a magic potion that it is marketed to be.

Many Americans are addicted to sweets. Sugar is subtly hidden in many of our foods, so even if we attempt to avoid sugar, you can consume large quantities of it in a multitude of food products. Children are the worst victims of hidden sugar; it is in all the foods advertised to children claiming to be beneficial to their good health. You will probably not find one food advertised to children that does not contain sugar. With their hyped names and brightly colored ingredients, TV commercials know how to pep the kids up on the most damagingly sweet cereals. It appears that sugar is only omitted from the diet when individuals are on a diet. While omitting sugar helps to lose weight, sugar has even more damaging effects than overweight, and certainly one main problem sugar creates is diabetes.

Sugar substitutes are readily used. One which health-minded individuals use is fructose; however, many are being fooled since this substitute is just as bad as sugar. A recent study released shows that fructose significantly raises triglyceride levels, which may increase the risk of heart disease. Americans are addicted to sweets of all kinds, and it is affecting them with a myriad of health problems. Some common sugar substitutes, available just about everywhere, are proven cancer causers.

Another supplement touted by health practitioners which does not live up its reputation is shark cartilage. The hyperbole about shark cartilage began with the concept that since sharks do not get cancer then this supplement must be effective for curing cancer in humans. This is a simplistic way of evaluating this concept. The Cancer Research Foundation, a non-profit research organization, came out with a report which pulls the rug from under shark cartilage, and thus caused much disappointment for those desperately looking for any form of cancer cure. Sixty patients with advanced cancer who were given shark cartilage and took no other form of cancer treatment were followed for ten months; shark cartilage was found to be ineffective. Patients were given huge doses of shark cartilage dissolved in water. To get the equivalent in the capsule form, that is usually the way this supplement is taken, would require taking 100 or more of 500 mg capsules daily and would cost thousands of dollars a month. These researchers cannot be accused of under-treating these patients, as can occur with researchers, because the patients were given mega-doses of shark cartilage; it appears this particular research was more than objective in its approach. As stated before, the results showed no benefit in taking shark cartilage. About twenty different doctors all agreed shark cartilage did not fit the bill and even worse, when patients blindly believed in its cure, the supplement may have curtailed other natural cancer cures…there are many.

Another supplement that has been highly hyped is MGN-3, in which the manufacturer claims its product is a "magic bullet" for curing cancer. Now this just adds another promise of cure to the multitude of cures out in the market. It appears that every day another promise is added to the list. MGN-3 is supposed to be a great cure because it increases the blood level of natural killer cells, white blood cells (leukocytes), in laboratory tests. The problem is there is no evidence it reduces tumor size. The manufacturers of this supplement are committing an illegal act, because they are making statements that it is a cancer cure and it has been proven that it is not a cancer cure. They have gotten away with it and the FDA has been very lax in allowing this to go on since it is illegal for any claims to be made for cancer cure unless approved by them. There is no harm in offering advice in preventing cancer, as long it is not touted as a promise for a cure.

Many alternative doctors are involved with cancer patients; however, their roles are to help slow down the cancer spread, make the patient comfortable, and teach them how to live with the affliction. One thing these natural health people avoid is the use of chemotherapy, since this treatment kills good cells, bad cells and every other cell it contacts. Chemotherapy makes patients even sicker and destroys their immune system. The end result of chemotherapy is…you will get very sick and then die. The end result for doctors who prescribe chemotherapy for patients with cancer is…you will get a lot of money, buy a new home and send your children to college. Are you getting an inkling why this dangerous chemotherapy is prescribed to patients with cancer? If that is not the reason for the extensive prescriptions of chemotherapy for patients with cancer, then the only other explanation is…doctors are not keeping current in their field or they refuse to consider alternative treatments that actually have proven to cure cancer.

WORKOUT

The following offers information on taking supplements: Remember, it is always best to consult a health practitioner or a nutritionist before taking any supplements. Carefully read directions before taking. Some vitamins and herbs are best taken at meals rather than on an empty stomach. Keep all supplements and herbs in a cool place, but most do not need to be refrigerated. Keep caps tightly shut. Purchase all your health products through reputable places, such as health food stores or through certain distributors, which are available through Dr. James F. Balch's health encyclopedia called *Nutritional Healing*. Products bought through grocery stores or pharmacies are, most often, less expensive and lack quality and are less effective, and have fillers, thus have less pure ingredients.

You will find listed on most supplements warning signs for pregnant women or those with special problems, to consult a physician prior to taking. Pay attention and follow the directions on "how much" and "how often" to take the supplement. Always take supplements and herbs with a full glass of water. (Note: Most herbs are strengthened with alcoholic beverages, so take less if you drink wine with your meals.) Keep track of how you are taking your supplements, and the quantity and length of time you are taking them; ensuring you get the most benefits from the herb or supplement. It usually requires several months to obtain full benefits, but you should see good results within about six weeks or less. If you do not start seeing results, good or bad, from an herb in about a week, you could be taking the wrong herb or supplement. Most herbs will let you know almost immediately if they are right for you...pay attention and do not hesitate in informing your practitioner what you are experiencing. Keep in reserve, and perhaps increase the dosage of certain vitamins only when you come down with particular problems, such as a sinus infection, colds or flus, indigestion, constipation, etc. You do not want to be taking a regimen of vitamins that will only function when you have a particular health problem...that could be unhealthy and hinder, or render ineffective, the supplement you take for the problem. Get advice from your health practitioner or health books written by known or familiar alternative medical physicians. Again, you cannot go wrong with Dr. Balch's most comprehensive health book. It will point you in the right direction and when your knowledge increases, you resources will increase.

Getting an excellent multivitamin is vital; it should have all the vitamins and minerals your body needs. My two favorites are "Allone" Nutritech from Santa Barbara, CA, tel.: 800-235-5727 and website, www. all-one.com. Since this product comes in powder form, you need to request a particular shaker or use your blender. For those who prefer the pill form, Dr. David Williams' Daily Advantage, a multi-nutrient supplement, provides it. It comes in packets which contain essential vitamins and minerals for supporting every function in your body, including eyesight, memory, circulation, and mobility. This product also contains advanced antioxidants, also EFA Advantage for cholesterol control, promotes normal blood pressure, and Herbal Super Food Booster, which promotes a peak immune system. I get my supply sent monthly and take two packets daily.

It is best to get on a regime where you take your supplements on a consistent and regular basis. Also, get a quality alternative health practitioner to examine you and then he or she can determine what would be best for you. You want to refrain from overdosing and taking supplements that you do not need. There are numerous herbal healing books on the market and specialists in the herbal and healing field whose advice will be beneficial to you. This manual covers most of these subjects.

STRINGENT CONTROLS

Provoked by the spread of the alternative healing movement, some physicians had gone so far as accusing those practicing alternative healing as being fraudsters or fanatics, and cautioned their patients of their possible harm. One standard scare tactic used is the warning that healing practices were not approved by the FDA.

Even further, the medical establishment teamed up with the powerful FDA, and for years, attempted to curtail the alternative healing movement with mantra. One such episode included wiping health supplements off the shelves of health stores and burying them under stringent controls of the medical establishment. Vitamins and herbs would be chained within the domain of medical doctors, and available only through prescriptions. When hints of this act started to emerge, enough people enthusiastically signed petitions against what they considered to be a dictatorial act...and won. Of course, there is never a guarantee that health supplements will continually be available to the public. The threat of supplements being confiscated due to possible criticism as being dangerous still remains. All that is needed is a few dissatisfied consumers making claims of negative side effects experienced from a particular supplement to perpetuate an investigation, even if such complaints are far from proving anything. One minor unproven incident can generate immediate cause for those anxious to be rid of any facets of natural healing to point their finger at its potential perils and demand it be removed from the shelves. Then of course, the FDA having the last word could eventually curtail sales of all supplements. Recently, the FDA was questioned for some of its negligence in permitting death-threatening pharmaceutical drugs to go on the market. In the meantime, many prayed that supplements would remain available, but it is truly surprising certain actions have not taken place yet. Though conscientious consumers have fought for free access to supplements, nothing permanent is stopping the FDA from trying the same thing again and using a minute negative incident to rationalize their action.

ACTIONS THAT CAN BE TAKEN TO ENSURE CONSUMER RIGHTS

Becoming aware of what can be done to curtail any action regarding the confiscation of supplements from the public; the public has a right to defend themselves against any denial of freedom in purchasing supplements and herbal remedies.

Supporting local health stores when they are faced with such threats; signing petitions against such enactments.

Using the Internet to contact others willing to join possible protest projects against the FDA; those fearing such an action can stock up on their favorite supplements and herbs. Expiration dates and proper storage conditions need to be accounted for.

Discussing this potential problem with alternative practitioners and others in the natural health field...see what steps can be taken to ensure consumers' rights to have these products available without a prescription.

CHAPTER 23

THE WHOLE-BEING CONNECTION

Medical science is on the threshold of understanding how emotional attitudes affect physical well-being. Research indicates that negative emotions are not just limited to causing high blood pressure and other stress-related afflictions, but can be responsible for manifesting chronic illnesses and even life-threatening diseases. Today's alternative healing seeking a wider spectrum of insights as to causes of illnesses takes this factor into account. It recognizes many physical ailments derive from emotional dysfunction and have cited that numerous individuals suffering from certain ailments fail to find relief from their family physicians simply because they are being treated from a narrow perspective, where emotions, in relation to physical well-being, are not considered in any healing process. To go further, certain ailments such as allergies, arthritis, even cancer, and a string of other physical problems affect those with emotional disorders more so than individuals experiencing mental well-being, and those with tendencies towards negative personalities suffer more from chronic ailments than individuals with positive outlooks.

A study made in 1982 at Johns Hopkins clinic for outpatients concluded that patients suffering depression, anxiety and other mental disorders took longer to heal than those in a positive frame of mind. Also discovered was that those with strong religious convictions healed more rapidly and their stays at the hospital were shorter and some of this rapid recovery was considered miraculous. Other researchers are making discoveries pertaining to the mind as being a vital factor in recovering from even deadly diseases.

The idea gains weight from new medical evidence that proves the mind actually influences our level of immunity. Researchers recently monitored the immune function of twenty ovarian cancer patients as they underwent monthly chemotherapy at Memorial Sloan-Kettering Cancer Center in New York City. They measured T cells, which are detrimental to substances in the body, in samples of blood taken at home several days prior to the treatments and in those taken in individuals entering the hospital for their treatment. The researchers discovered that the immune system functions were suppressed in the hospital... their healing slowed down. Upon entering the hospital, the patients became nauseated prior to chemotherapy. It was determined that the subjects were experiencing some sort of conditioned response that was responsible for suppressing their immune system.

Another factor regarding the power of the mind over the body is evident in the key to longevity. This key to physical deterioration from old age is not derived from physical means but from the brain and the protein deterioration on your string DNA. Various scientific factors are involved in the brain, such as neurotransmitters and hormones, such as dopamine, acetylcholine and estrogen, all of which are part of the signal-transduction system that gives cells the go-ahead to proceed. As we age, receptors for some of these substances become weakened or sparse in certain parts of the body. With proper diet, exercise and stress reduction, and most important mind stimulation, these receptors can remain strong and young. Even more important is the realization that longevity is not bound by physical aging but from one's attitude and self-awareness, which can act as preventive measures against aging.

LIFE FORCE

For many years, individual scientists, physiologists and biologists have suspected that each person had within him/her some universal energy or vitality that motivates the human machine. The amount of energy and how it was utilized determines how certain individuals are more resistant to disease than others are; why some age faster than others and why some hardy people live longer than others do. Further research has determined that "universal energy" goes beyond the surface of the human body, and is derived from proper nutrition and lifestyle. It is true that a certain degree of energy is derived physiologically from nutrients of food and air, but clinical psychologists have claimed that also in the workings, perhaps even more powerful, that a source of power regarded as "impulse" works through us. This "mental energy" is believed to be a force which ebbs and flows in healthy individuals. This view suggests we are more than receptacles, we are channels of energy. In other words, life and power are not so much contained in us, but through us.

J. A. Hadfield mentioned in his *The Psychology of Power* whether we look at this as cosmic energy, as a life force, or what may be its relation to the Divine Immanence in Nature, is still a mystery, but one that could be very real. Today, further study has established this "life source" as scientific fact. Dr. Hans Seyle of the University of Montreal focused on what he believed to be the deterrent factor in health maintenance, which he claimed was stress. Clinically, and in numerous laboratory experiments and studies, Dr. Seyle proved the existence of a basic life force, which he called "adaptation energy."

Throughout life, from cradle to the grave, we are called upon to "adapt" to stress situations. Even the process of just existing constitutes stress and brings up the continual need for adaptation. In his studies, he discovered the human body contains various natural defense mechanisms, local adaptation syndromes or L.A.S., its function being to defend against specific stress, and a general defense mechanism, general adaptation syndrome or G.A.S., which defends against nonspecific stress. In this situation, the term "stress" means any change which requires adaptation or adjustment, such as extremes of hot or cold, invasion by disease germs, emotional tension, the wear and tear of living or the so-called "aging process."

TRICKS OF THE SUBCONSCIOUS MIND

A recent study on attitudes discovered that serious illness, and even accidents, could result from a negative attitude. Depression, which not only is a major cause of chronic fatigue, allergies, migraine headaches, and backaches, can even cause self-afflicted accidents. An individual with a death wish, but lacking courage to commit suicide, entertains a certain subliminal message and transmits that message to their unconscious mind, causing this message to be carried out by the manifestation of a life- threatening illness or even from what may appear as a freak accident.

Individuals suffering from a guilty conscience can manifest a subconscious message which initiates some sort of self-punishment. This sense of unconscious self-retribution goes unnoticed by the individual but what is happening is the subconscious mind in this digressive state, attempts to sort out imbalanced negativities, causing individuals to unknowingly neglect their safety valve of self-survival (or the will to love), thus magnifying their vulnerability to negative occurrences. This mental digression can result in lowering normal cautionary measures of survival where the individual is more prone to accept potentially dangerous and self-destructive conditions; under normal circumstances, the person would avoid these dangers.

Mental therapists report that the subconscious mind is a powerful thing, and it plays an active role in your everyday life. At the same time, its potential of self-destruction can be extremely obscure and subtle. Conflicts emerging in the subconscious mind can manifest self-afflictions of all sorts, from occurrences of illness to life-threatening accidents. On the other hand, those with an enormous will to live can undergo a multitude of precarious conditions with minimal ill effects. How often do we hear of seemingly fatal illnesses miraculously cured, only to discover that the afflicted individual was endowed with an extremely positive attitude? This positive reverence for life develops a potent defensive force that is able to will the illness away. In the meantime, while some may give credence to the occurrence of these phenomena, to some sort of underlining spiritual entity, perhaps a more down-to-earth rationale explains that attitude plays an extremely vital role in keeping healthy and fit, others dismiss it as non-existing. A profound indication of emotions affecting physical conditions is evident where bereaving mourners, after the death of a lifetime spouse, may die shortly after, and often referred to as *"dying from a broken heart."* Such a terminology leaves the medical scientific community baffled, since death from a broken heart is medically impossible.

We can conclude that mental attitudes are the controlling factor over much of our lives, and that our level of physical well-being is determined by our outlook on life. A recent report given at a meeting of the American Heart Association in New Orleans claimed that an individual could reverse artery blockage by attitudes and lifestyles changes. In people with blocked coronary arteries, while adhering to a strict vegetarian diet, engage in daily mild exercise, the practice of stress-reduction and maintaining positive attitudes is even more vital and can actually reverse the blockage. This study also found that change in diet and exercise alone were not enough to reverse heart disease and that healthy mental attitude is a more important factor than has been generally recognized by heart specialists.

A 1990 study at Johns Hopkins Hospital by Dr. Mark Luskin reported how certain lifestyle conditions affected physical health. His conclusion was that, of those individuals prone to frequent accidents and chronic physical problems, such as backaches, migraine headaches, allergies, diabetes, high blood pressure, and other illnesses, over seventy percent experienced some type of disruptive well-being. Some of these individuals were undergoing divorces, were discontent in their work, dissatisfied with their life in general, living with abusive spouses, or not able to let go of childhood problems.

Physical ailments caused from mental attitudes can be observed in how mental stress can provoke various physical deteriorations, such as heart disease, cancer, allergies, ulcers, chronic fatigue as well as many other afflictions. The connection between mental and physical exists with patients suffering from hypochondria. These chronic health complainers often use poor health as a defense mechanism or as a means of crying out for attention. Studies have shown people suffering from this disease are often exposed to unsympathetic environments, where such emotions as the craving for love and care often go unnoticed. Consequently, prolonged ignored appeals eventually manifest themselves into physical ailments. When a sound diagnosis cannot be defined, the ailment is placed in the illusive category of hypochondria; however, for the patient, this lack of well-being is very real; they know they are not feeling well.

TESTIMONIAL

One situation showing how emotions affect physical chronic ailments pertains to a young woman named Susan. Susan is a hypochondriac; she is a chronic complainer of physical ailments. These ailments only occur when she is in the company of her mother, who is a domineering person. One day Susan met her mother for lunch and was feeling fine; soon after her mother arrived, Susan immediately started to feel ill and complained of a stomachache and nausea. When her mother left the luncheon, Susan started feeling better. Susan came to understand that these sudden attacks of illnesses occurred only when she was in the presence of her mother. She also came to understand her deep resentment towards her mother, which she could not openly express, was manifested in the form of a physical ailment.

Here we see a relationship between the mind and physical well-being. If Susan were seeking a cure, she would immediately focus on her physical problem and go see a physician. Unaware of the relationship between her physical ailments and her emotional ailments, she did not consider the cure of the physical being in the realm of the emotional.

Alternative healing does not make separate distinction between emotional and physical well-being; patients suffering from hypochondria are diagnosed as suffering from some emotional problem. Getting down to the potential emotional underlying cause of physical illness helps patients to become more aware, perhaps of the root of their health issues and see the relationship to their emotional well-being and from there proceed with self-healing thorough obtaining positive attitudes. Knowing that one's mind is responsible for causing a physical problem most often is enough to get onto the road to recovery; no one wishes to be sick, not even hypochondriacs. While these patients resolve their problems, they may use diverse reactions towards resolving similar feelings, such as anger, in which aggressiveness, even acts of violence will be the outcome.

BODY TALK

How many of us take the time to really talk to ourselves and take the initiative to probe into our subconscious mind to manifest some stuck well-hidden information that may offer a clue as to what is causing a particular health problem. In reality, we often seek out a medical person whenever suffering from a physical or mental problem rather than looking towards the power within ourselves to heal. Who knows better than ourselves the state of our emotions and physical health? When in a state of illnesses, we become more vulnerable and thus, lack the confidence in seeking our powers to heal ourselves. The expectations of alternative healing practitioners are having their patients take an active role in their healing process, and they motivate patients to seek out their own powers to self-heal. This can simply mean they take it upon themselves to follow certain health regimens to maintain good health. Body Talk is becoming a growing interest in the subject of self-healing. It is a terminology that refers to various healing modalities which include the process of seeking one's own inner strengths. Intuitive questioning is prompted by a Body Talk practitioner to reveal certain answers pertaining to self-healing. The best method of approaching this is through a period of meditation. If you are suffering from an emotional or physical ailment, you attempt searching for the relationship between cause and effect of this particular problem. Let's say you are suffering from a chronic illness, perhaps afflicting you for many years, and have tried all types of healing processes, both traditional and alternative, and still get no relief. The Body Talk practitioner helps the patient to "talk it out," so as to get to the underlying problem of the origin of the illnesses...be it physical or emotional. This "talk" differs from psychology therapy. Rather than initially focusing on the emotional and omitting physical concerns, this therapy uses both the emotional and physical well-being of the patient during the healing process; the premise being that the body can hold physical damages, perhaps stemming from past emotional wounds. It is believed that many illnesses stem from past physical and mental traumas that occurred in our childhood. If they are recognized and then understood, the present problem may be solved.

TESTIMONIAL

Alice Drew suffers chronic fatigue, which resulted in disabling her from work. Being hit by such a debilitating ailment after being healthy most of her life, Alice became depressed. As an aware person, she realized that emotional trauma might be responsible for her illness. She reflects on a very traumatic episode in her life she believes was responsible for her problem. She recalls how she became numb with fear when the building trembled where she worked, located beside the Pentagon during the 9/11 terrorist attack. This made a tremendous emotional impact on Alice, which may have manifested into a nervous disorder, which later on manifested into chronic fatigue. It took some time for her to piece together how certain emotions affect her health. She looked back to see what other traumas may have contributed to her sudden illness, considering the following were happening at the same time; she was out of a job, going through a divorce, her five children had grown and left home and now she felt useless, both as a career woman and as a mother. She concluded that collectively, all could be reasons for her physical downfall; however, at first, she unsuccessfully traveled the circuit of seeking healing from traditional methods, but the complexities relating to her situation made healing difficult and alternative healing means had to be sought out.

Body Talk was Alice's choice for healing. Her healing process started out with her being able to affirm to herself that it was alright to be out of a job and that her children no longer needed her, that neither was her fault. Self-forgiving is something that had not crossed her mind; not only did this woman feel useless, her pride in herself was crushed, and she felt disappointment to her family. Through Body Talk healing, Alice learned about the cause/effect of her illness. She no longer looked at her body in disgust, nor resented what happened to her. She learned in therapy how to talk to her body and ask for it to heal, and eventually it did.

OUR SENSES, OUR HEALTH

The practice of clinically dissecting of patients where technical applications become more important than the personality of the patient not only ignores the humanistic aspect of treatment but also proves to be an unsuccessful approach to healing. Rushed in and out of white sterile rooms flooded with acrid medicine fumes, patients are physically scrutinized in cold indifference, barely communicating with their attendants. This lack of contact between physicians and patients should not be taken lightly. While professionals may regard their patients' comments as small talk, it is through this vital communication that intricate nuances can be evaluated. The revealing of patients' mental attitudes is critical in offering insight into the cause of obscure chronic states of physical ailments. We are aware the effects of stress, anxiety and depression have on physical well-being; medical treatments are not complete until the mental state of the patient is taken into account.

SUMMARY

1—Emotions can be a powerful source for healing as well as a powerful destroyer.

2—Attitudes can cause physical and mental conflicts as well as act as a source of healing.

3—The mind, body and spirit are related and affect the other, all three need treatment when illness occurs.

WORKOUT

Study the following...

1—Always attempt to connect cause and effect in any of your behavioral patterns to your physical health. This list reveals how certain emotional problems can have an effect on your physical health and help you to become aware of the precise causes responsible for certain problems. Awareness of cause and effect, how your mental attitude can be responsible for any possible physical ailments, gives you the whole picture of any given situation and empowers you to take more control over your own health.

2—Listing times when you feel stress will have an effect on your physical well-being. Studies show that colds, fever blisters, cold sores, mouth cankers, flue and other ailments tend to increase when any form of stress is experienced; students just prior to taking major tests that determine their career status, or loss of a loved one, losing a job, etc., suffer more from the above-listed ailments. It is advisable that at these times of stress you pay close attention and adhere to the following: maintain a good diet and exercise, get plenty of sleep and relaxation, calm your mind and carefully work your way through the cause of the stress or anxiety or if the cause of the stress is unknown, calmly seek its cause.

List some "cause and effects" pertaining to your present mental mood; if you feel listless, unmotivated, or perhaps restless, the following may be the cause: lack of exercise, feeling of not accomplishing your worthwhile goals, or having a guilty conscience…you may be experiencing difficulty accepting something you did.

3—If you are suffering from depression, observe how it affects your physical health, such as lowering your immune system, causing body aches and pains, oversleeping, overeating, and getting into various conflicts. In your times of happiness and contentment, make the same observations when you were depressed.

KEEPING ACTIVE

For Emotional, Mental and Physical Well-Being

> *As we pump that iron, our brain cells swell,*
> *Aggressions are released and all is well.*

When we think of any form of bodily exercise, usually what comes to mind is exercising for losing weight or for bodybuilding. Attitudes towards exercise have changed. Exercise is now considered as a tool for deep relaxation of the mind and body and such intrinsic values as a growing awareness of one's body. As for basic health benefits, medical scientific evidence shows that many major illnesses benefit from daily exercise, such as diabetes, cholesterol, heart disease, circulatory problems and the list goes on. Doctors are now prescribing weightlifting for those suffering from osteoporosis; also good for arthritis are stretching exercises. Different forms of exercise, such as yoga, are excellent for alleviating stress, excellent for keeping the body toned and flexible, and tai chi, an ancient Eastern body-mind practice, for developing good balance and inner peace.

Western science is discovering what the East has believed for centuries...that mind-body exercise I powerful medicine. With America's recent awakening to the mind-body connection, the pounding aerobics and jogging boom begun in the 1960s has evolved into a host of more gentle beneficial practices. Today, mind-body fitness disciplines permeate community fitness programs, gyms and wellness centers. They are being instituted in rehabilitation facilities and even medical offices. Healing physical practices, such as hatha yoga, tai chi and Pilates, have gained the most attention and are offered in exercise gyms that just a few years ago would never dream of offering such lofty types of exercises. Now these centers are regarded as being more than just bodybuilding entities, they are places that welcome various forms of mind-body healing and where individuals can overcome injuries, tend to their own physical therapy needs and with the assistance of professional trainers, who are becoming more proficient in the treatment of body ailments, are enjoying better health. People see improved coordination and daily functioning as they discover how the mind, body, and spirit play together to make life better in every way.

The mind can transform muscles beyond what pure movement can do; that is why athletes concentrate, dancers focus, and mind-body fitness enthusiasts meditate. With many yoga-type classes, meditation is part of the training and movement transforms thinking, manifest in fresh ideas and insights. Thoreau, Plato, Einstein and Wordsworth regularly took long walks to gain insight to problems and to develop creative ideas. Physical fitness, in any of its forms, makes you feel good and look better, but it is so much more…it is rewarding and healing to deepen the experience beyond an external shift in strength and shape to lasting inner and outer well-being. Mind-body fitness delivers the gains of traditional exercise without the pain and strain on the body, which in itself, can have damaging repercussions. With healing exercise, more gentle contemplative practices actually relax the body while opening mental pathways to one's spiritual and emotional growth as well as healing physical afflictions.

Ralph LaForge, a clinical exercise physiologist with Duke University, put it this way regarding mind-body exercise, "Think of the output as creativity, clarity and enriched physical and emotional health." LaForge served as the technical reviewer or *Mind-Body Fitness for Dummies*, a user- friendly introductory manual authored by Therese Iknoian, president of Total Fitness Network. In her book, she mentions that flowing routines of meditative awareness practices consistently applied result in obtaining a peaceful calm and centered confidence that translate to all aspects of life. Daily tasks become more manageable, where stressful situations become minimized. Such form of exercise energizes and helps one to focus better. It also enhances a meditative spiritual attitude towards life in general where one, while in slow contemplative movements, can generate a feeling of balance and become centered with the universe. While in motion, concentration is focused on each part of the body where one can notice which parts are weakest or strongest and then carefully take note how the body is being healed through individual movements and exercises. The following are three of the most basic mind-body exercises:

1—HATHA YOGA—One of the multitudes of yoga disciplines— benefits are extreme stretching, flexibility, giving balance to the body and mind. Each position is involved with contemplative concentration and awareness in breathing and in thought. Yoga keeps muscles elongated while helping to relax them. Yoga helps to maintain mind and body awareness where the individual feels more in control over their being. With this, daily bodily and mental activities are not taken for granted, but controlled.

2—TAI CHI—is one form of Chinese martial arts in which orchestrated movements free the flow of omnipotent omnipresent energy through the body. Experiencing this energy yields more health, happiness and peace. Tai chi's credo is "go slow and slower still, as slow as humanly possible." Fitness is not the goal here but deep relaxation, breath control, and balance are predominant interests in this beautiful ancient practice. Tai chi is beneficial for several health problems. The first predominant benefit is deep meditation and concentration while in motion. Since the movements are rather complex, it requires thought, since instruction during a session are not given, instead individuals have to follow along while the instructor is doing the movements. Tai chi also is excellent for exercising the memory and is particularly beneficial for the elderly. People with Parkinson can find the benefits of this practice because it helps with balance and flexibility, which is a particular concern with this disease. As for the deep relaxation aspect resulting from tai chi, stress reduction is helpful for those with high blood pressure and heart disease. What appears to be a moderate form of exercise truly is an excellent means of healing some very vital health concerns.

Westerners' idea of exercise for health, for many years, has been weightlifting. As little as a few years ago, yoga or tai chi would have been considered too exotic for the average American health spa and not acceptable to most spa members. That trend has changed and these exercises have become the norm in most gyms. Rather than blaring music, the pounding of feet and the sound of weights being dropped on the gym floor, soft music permeates dim-lit rooms and barely a word can be heard.

3—PILATES—has been introduced in health spas relatively recently. It is a structured system of small isolated movements that demands powerful focus on feeling every nuance of muscle action while working out on the floor mats or machines. Softer than traditional exercises, Pilates, like yoga, yields long, lean, flexible muscles. Lithe, limber and gracefully balanced movements readily translate to everyday activities;

walking, sitting and bending helps overcome injuries. Instructors focus on developing the torso's abdominal power center through mental mastery. The more focused, the fewer repetitions are needed.

The Feldenkrais method helps students straighten out what founder Moshe Feldenkrais calls "kinks in your brain." Kinks are learned movement patterns that no longer serve. They may have been adopted to compensate for a physical or emotional injury or to accommodate individuality in the social world. Students unlearn unworkable movements and discover better-personalized ways to move. Benefits apply to everything from rising out of bed, sitting in a chair, opening a jar, to athletic activities. Benefits include better circulation and digestion, increased self-confidence, alertness, fewer headaches and backaches and sleep that is more restful.

The Alexander technique in Pilates teaches the correct way of doing daily movements, from brushing your teeth to holding a knife, standing in line, working on a computer, how to pick up light and heavy objects, how to correctly reach for items on high shelves and any other habit which may be causing particular body aches and pains. The technique also teaches how to prevent future problems. It is believed each crook of a toe or finger may reflect something else that is going on in the body. According to the Alexander technique, nearly everyone has an unhealthy relationship between his or her head and neck and it is revealed in how they carry themselves. The point is not to just work out the heart, lungs, muscles, mind and body but to facilitate a more effective workout for organs, muscles and bones.

Medical studies tend to lack information on the healing aspect of mind- body exercise but now it is coming more into play due to the diversity of data confirming the benefits of exercise in healing all sorts of illnesses. While just about everyone recognizes that such exercises as running, walking, swimming and gym workouts are excellent means of maintaining health, few recognize that adding "mindful" exercise is even more beneficial. Many professionals believe that "mindful" is even more effective in alleviating high blood pressure, lowering cholesterol, alleviating chronic pain, helping to prevent falls and reducing anxiety and stress. Persistent practice of Pilates exercise has additional benefits, increasing endurance, strengthening the immune system, strengthening the heart and lung system plus developing muscle and bone strength as well as adding flexibility and balance.

HARD WORK AND HEALTH

Dr. Dean Ornish of the Preventive Medicine Research Institute in Sausalito, California, and a colleague at the University of California at San Francisco and the University of Texas Medical School in Houston, did a medical study which included questioning why some competitive hard- driving people end up with coronary heart disease while others live long healthy lives. In recent studies, a test was made regarding 150 middle-aged males over a ten-year period. At the outset, fifty had heart disease, fifty reported high risk factors (smoking, high blood pressure and cholesterol), and fifty had neither. Each man was classified as either a hard-driving Type A or an easy-going Type B. Researchers measured the frequency of "recreational social activities" like entertaining friends, playing games, involvement with craft projects, attending parties and sports events. Surprisingly, after ten years, the mortality rates for Type-A and Type-B men were similar, despite the active Type-A men being more vulnerable to heart disease.

The most important find was that the mortality rate of hard-driving men decreased when they were involved with social activities. This included the focus on healthy ambitions and positive attitudes. This research concluded that when the same group of men became hostile or angry, their risk of heart disease increased, because the researchers selected this group of men to experience different stresses. Contrary to popular belief, stress is more prevalent in hard-driving, hardworking people; this research concluded that ambition and hard work is beneficial and that coronary heart disease was the result of unsocial behavior and aggressiveness.

Now that more women are acquiring prestigious careers, putting more energy and time into their work, their domestic issues increased. This is an added load of stress and most likely responsible for causing chronic fatigue syndrome, which has been labeled a women's disease.

Reports indicate that it is not just the high-level workload involved here but it is psychological factors leading the way, the same psychological factors their equivalent high-ranking males experience. If a woman has problems accepting her career over her family needs, her feelings of guilt may result in such maladies as chronic migraine headaches and ulcers. She may also become depressed, which can affect her career and in turn result in inner conflicts of her priorities.

While we may regard work as a cause of stress for some women, their accomplishments keep them mentally healthy. No doubt, there is some truth to work-related stress, but in general, productive occupations, where the mind immerses itself in interesting endeavors are fuels that keep the mind active, content and healthy. Dr. Brenda B. Toner observed indicators of the relationship between emotional and physical health in a study conducted by her and colleagues at the Clark Institute of Psychiatry in Toronto called the "Irritable Bowel Syndrome." This study is all conclusive in part, that emotions play an active role in the physical health of individuals. IBS, the scientific term for this condition, is prevalent with fast-track baby boomers. Tests show women suffering from IBS had symptoms of poor sleeping and bad appetites, lethargy or feelings of hopelessness and helplessness, gastric problems, suppression of feelings, where they were denied or ignored, and in need for individual self-image improvements, as well as the desire to show good impressions to others, could often churn up the gastric system, causing stress, anxiety and depressions. When feelings could be expressed and honestly focused on, such symptoms were often alleviated, even when the patient's emotional problems were still evident.

Answer the following:

WORKOUT

1—Have you been able to detect a particular connection between your mental well-being with a particular ailment?

2—When you are under stress, does a particular chronic pain bother you more?

3—Do you feel physically better when on vacation, away from work, or just having a good time?

4—Do you feel physically better when working?

5—Evaluate how certain individuals, situations or places affect you mentally or physically and then do you know the reason why?

6—Do you suffer from a chronic condition that you think you can attribute to some emotional problem now or in your past?

Treating patients with their mental well-being in mind is not revolutionary. In the past, family physicians were not only responsible for their patients' physical health but emotional well-being. They often were friends of the family, offering warm psychological advice, lecturing on the evils of too much alcohol and just generally expressing a personal interest towards those under their care.

HELPFUL HINTS

Since alternative healing practitioners are growing in number, specific names are not included. Listed below is information that will help you find the right healer that will best represent your condition:

1—You need to search for a practitioner who integrates emotional well-being with physical ailments and does not separate the two; even better is a healer who focuses on spiritual healing. The "offered therapies" should focus on the possibility that emotional dysfunctions could be the cause, or at least related to the physical afflictions, and the therapy needs to address the two simultaneously.

2—You need to feel free to ask your physician questions. Even today, many physicians vehemently separate emotional issues when tending to a patient's physical problems. Make sure you are comfortable with the person from whom you are seeking treatment, and that physician is patient and willing to discuss your health problems prior to making an appointment. (You may determine that the treatment offered is inappropriate or unacceptable to your needs.)

3—Nothing is more discouraging than when a natural healing practitioner shows characteristics associated with allopathic healers and the "medical establishment." Things to watch for in your natural healing practitioner (homeopathic healer) that would indicate their lack of knowledge or interest in your case include being too clinical, minimizing discussions, impatient or inflexible (rigid) in their evaluation or a hurried interest to refer you to another practitioner. That is not the kind of practitioner you want healing your maladies. Above all, you must trust and have faith in the healer you choose…this is critical if you want to heal.

4—Any treatment, particularly for chronic illnesses, requires much faith in the healer who practices mind-body-spirit therapies because first of all, you will be dealing with unfamiliar healing techniques, and second, usually such therapies require longer periods of time for the healing process to manifest itself. Holistic healing, unlike conventional medical treatment, treats the mental and physical human, and since you need time to heal, you need to develop a good trusting relationship with your realer. To acquire the most effective result from healing therapies, you need a positive attitude at all times, both between your healer and you and with yourself.

5—As mentioned in the previous chapter, check out credentials. This may be a bit difficult since you are searching in some unfamiliar territories; word of mouth, local healing associations and groups can be your starting point. Get references and testimonials from other patients. Check up on the particular associations the practitioner claims to belong, then check up on the association, find out exactly what they do, what is their main purpose and contributions they have made in healing, what are their philosophies about healing, and familiarize yourself with their members and the member who directed to you this particular healer. Check their educational background, special studies and the particular type of healing in which they specialized. You may discover along the way that certain prominent names come up in your reference checking, such as Dr. Andrew Weil, Dr. Wayne Dyer, Dr. Gary Null, etc. All of these doctors treat their patients with the realized importance of the individual's emotions and spiritual life.

6—Remember that most of these treatments and expenses will be "out of pocket." Some health professionals are willing to arrange payment according to the individual's ability to pay.

7—Since the medical community does not recognize alternative medicine, take caution prior to commitment with whom you choose to render treatment. Recently there has been a rash of medical doctors who are integrating holistic medicine in their prescription regime. These individuals are combining some of their professional knowledge with new modes of health, thus you get the benefits of both the homeopathic and allopathic miracles. As medical doctors tend to lean towards treating physical ailments and minimize the mental and spiritual aspect of healing…you want to search for a practitioner who balances out the healing of the mind, body and spirit.

MORE UNDERSTANDING

Understanding the connection between the mind, body and spirit, along with those in the health fields minimizing technological dominance usage on patients, and the ones beginning to initiate alternative innovative methods of healing, such as incorporating concern and compassion in their treatment, will help advance the medical field as a whole. While such pioneer medical concepts may prove threatening to those who look to stringent rules of science to diagnose illnesses, changes are rippling throughout various holistic centers, who have taken the lead in focusing on the concept of the mind-body connection. The result of this rapid convergence means that people will receive better care from their practitioners with shorter healing time and less harmful side effects. Many lifetime sufferers have failed to receive relief for their medical ailments for the basic reason that they have not connected their mental attitude with their physical problems. Many cases report chronic ailment alleviation with the help of alternative medicines. A change made to lifestyles shows that positive lifestyle changes and a positive attitude implemented into their spiritual healing has performed "miracles" with these lifetime sufferers of chronic ailments. Several alternative spiritual centers offer courses on "miracles" where members pray for each other and the results are often miraculous.

CHAPTER 24

EMOTIONS AND HEALTH

GRIEF AND HEALTH

There are several "new-age" live-in centers offering healing programs for people experiencing grief. One particular center called Serenity House is located in the beautiful rolling hills of Maryland. This peaceful countryside sanctuary offers a temporary abode, particularly beneficial for those in the climax of their grief. Its distinctive spiritual ambience derives from the combination of the rural mountainous surroundings and the center's careful planning of activities and programs. This center is embraced by the governing, but caressing hands, of a free-spirited Catholic nun, Sister Katherine McGanus, who also is chairwoman of the humanities department at Loyola College, who just happens to never follow speed limits both in driving and in life.

Daily activities include yoga exercises, along with meditative/ spiritual prayers throughout the day. Included are renowned speakers discussing issues regarding health and well-being and a series of workshops on various healing processes. Particular attention is given to methods in health prevention, such as maintaining good physical and emotional health, particularly needed for those suffering depression and stress- related problems. This includes following highly nutritional menus and daily exercising, such as sunrise hikes, which can include a five-mile hike taking place at the break of dawn. Other beneficial activities include working in the center's "garden of life," a plot of herbs and organic vegetables, managed by a very old Chinese gardener and herbalist, where members can get their hands in the soil, at the same time planting the center's vegetables and herbs which are used for nutritional and medicinal healing. Such daily physical activity also helps to cure insomnia, a prevalent problem with those suffering grief.

Such a place can be an extreme turning point for some individuals, changing their lives forever, while to others it may prove very challenging. It is difficult for some to transform from a highly stressful executive position and conform to a low-key environment, but by the time such individuals resort to entering Serenity House, they are prepared to make these drastic changes. At first, the most pronounced alteration of a day's activities, and perhaps the most difficult, includes individuals learning to get in tune with their being. This means slowing down to a turtle's pace so you can learn to enjoy the here and now, and to learn how to savor and appreciate each moment, which is an excellent recipe for stress reduction.

Although it has been discovered that clinical depression is treatable, certain clinical treatments use methods which can be more harmful than beneficial. Two treatments commonly used are antidepressant medications and electroshock therapy, both of which can have adverse side effects. Psychotherapy is another method used but only serves as a Band-Aid to temporarily relieve the problem. Its side effect...it takes a considerably long time for the treatment to work. The various methods used in alternative healing to treat depression and grief are not only more effective but help to instill certain positive habits that can function for a lifetime. With the workshops and lectures offered on how to rid the body and mind of negative habits, negative emotions, learning stress-releasing skills, practicing daily meditation, involvement with productive activities, even change in diet, and adherence to some form physical activity, and spending time with nature all contribute to the many miraculous healing results. For some, Serenity House serves as a haven and it becomes stressful for those having to leave.

ATTITUDE AND HEALING

Sally was only seven when he encountered near death and as a neglected orphan, her illnesses went untreated until she got a severe case of pneumonia. In her hospital bed, Sally overheard a doctor comment, "I don't think she will make it." It appeared no one really cared if she did, but someone did. A compassionate nurse took a personal interest in Sally, carefully tending over her, picking a pattern for a nightgown she planned to make for the girl with her own hands. Sally was given hope and more important, "care." Knowing Sally had no parents, the nurse visited her on a daily basis, acting like a loving mother. Gradually, Sally regained her strength and in no time returned to a normal healthy girl.

Psychosomatic illness is more prevalent than we realize. A mother raising children, or tending after a sick husband, will not allow herself to get sick. It is as though she has "willed" herself to remain well so she can attend to their needs. One situation included a mother in her forties who had raised five children and also held down a job. After the last nineteen- year-old boy moved away from home this woman experienced a severe case of carpel tunnel syndrome, which left her hands and arms paralyzed. It was as though, after raising her children, she no longer was useful and subconsciously "willed" herself into becoming "useless." After going into counseling, she realized how much her husband needed her, and gradually she was able to rid her arms of the affliction.

Studies show that some women undergo severe depression and other debilitating diseases when their children grow up and leave home (the empty nest syndrome). Most women feeling that once their purpose in life is gone, such as raising their children, they have no meaningful reason to live. This can possibly lead to subconscious self-destruction, which often manifests in some form of illness. In the case where a spouse is responsible for taking care of his or her partner during illness, if one should die, often the other will die soon after. Some medical reports claim this is due to a "broken heart" or "lacking the will to live." In these scenarios, we can see how mental well-being plays a strong role in our lives, and even be responsible for the level of health we choose to maintain.

A MORE POSITIVE APPROACH TO HEALING

The practice of tribal shamanic healing has its basis on lifting the spirits of the sick and surrounding them with positive healing auras. Incantations and various spiritual enactments were devoted to patients, including giving him or her healing herbs and perhaps even hands-on-therapy…a wellness wish, all done under a positive attitude. The shaman believed that patients were in part responsible for their own recovery, and had the power to will themselves healed; some environments in which the sick recovered could be considered festive. The Southwest Hopi American Indians made beautiful bright-colored sand paintings for healing. The healing ceremony included soft repetitive chanting, similar to the lullabies we sing to calm our children, delivering a calming healing power over the patient. Some healing rituals included song and dance and various other ritualistic enactments to calm patients' spirits. The tribesmen believed this made the environment more conducive to healing. This differed enormously from the cold sterile environments Western hospitals offer their patients.

DEPRESSION AND MEMORY LOSS

Depression can be a reason for memory loss, perhaps the major cause. One of the greatest fears of a mental health patient is the fear of memory loss. The recent flood of information on Alzheimer's disease has made the public aware of the devastating deterioration it causes the brain. People become concerned when they experience any degree of memory loss, and they believe that the smallest memory loss is the first stage of this dreaded disease. People experience memory loss for a variety of reasons; most memory loss is treatable and even reversible. Perhaps the most common cause of memory loss and intellectual deterioration comes from what is termed "clinical depression" and not the "everyday blues." When deep depression is experienced, the loss of concentration develops, making it difficult for the affected person to acquire information. Even when certain data encodes in the brain, lack of concentration makes memory traces shallow. The "slowed-down thinking process" associated with depression makes the retrieval of memories more difficult.

Memory loss and depression often result from feelings of not being relevant or being part of the workings of life. Individuals who may, for many years, experience a high degree of success, then suddenly lose their status, gradually start feeling useless and unproductive and slump into depression. Those in management, or any type of leadership positions, can experience difficulties in letting go and when it is time for retirement, they can experience traumatic depression. In attempts to compensate for feelings of uselessness and loss of self-esteem, the retiree often expresses over-aggressive behavior and negative attitudes toward family members and others. Women or men with such spouses may find life unbearable and lack the ability to accept the spouse's retirement. Until this level of life is accepted, the individual is unable to find enjoyment in retirement. Depression seeping may cause memory loss and the individual blames this on "don't have to remember nothing now."

Memory loss can be corrected by self-help practice of more natural means. The simple act of correcting the diet can keep the memory more active. Numerous reports state that diets lacking an adequate amount of the B-complex vitamins, particularly thiamine, niacin and B-12, can produce dementia (brain disease with loss of memory). Thiamine deficiency is more apparent with alcohol abusers because they often do not eat properly. Severe lack of niacin, found in meats and fish, can lead to pellagra, which possess symptoms of memory loss. Severe anemia, which cuts down the amount of oxygen carried by the blood, can also causes memory loss.

While most people are aware that smoking can increase your chance of heart disease and lung ailments, there is inadequate information about the cause of brain diseases to place any blame on smoking tobacco. Severe chronic obstructive lung disease can lessen the amount of oxygen available to the brain; in fact, anything that interferes with oxygen going to the brain will decrease brain function. A good regimen of exercise helps to stimulate oxygen, thus more oxygen is able to flow to the brain. Since exercise can help release poisons in the body and get rid of them, oxygen in the body tends to be cleaner, thus giving more energy and vitality to the exerciser.

WHAT ABOUT YOU?

Comforting bedside manners is a concept far removed in today's technological healing methods. At one time, doctors relied on their nurses for intimate contact with patients that because of their busy schedules, they were unable to comfort or console. Today, highly technologically trained nurses, inundated with too many duties, have little incentive to employ such "bedside" duties. Patients rarely receive any extra attention from the doctor or nurse during the pre- or post-healing time. There is little said or even thought about the fact such negligence in bedside manners on the part of nurses and doctors have very negative effects on their patients.

Looking back, the old-fashioned house calls enabled physicians to offer individual attention to their patients. This included firsthand inspection of patients' convalescent surroundings, such as sanitary conditions, level of proper nourishment and just as important, social environmental situations. The doctor could observe family members' involvement in taking care of the patient. Patients in positive living conditions, surrounded by loving care, tend to recover from illness more rapidly than those living alone who suffer from longer-term illnesses resulting from loneliness and depression. Denied this wide scope of viewing patients, today's physicians have less comprehensive outlooks to work with.

In an attempt by the physician to arrive at a correct diagnosis, patients often have to resort to taking a series of costly tests. With a better holistic understanding of the patient, such as the patient's emotional well-being and living habits, the physician could enable the patient to assist in the diagnosis, thus rendering a more accurate diagnosis and enabling faster healing time.

At the same time, modern technology has supplied physicians' offices with high-tech medical equipment, rendering patients' ability to assist in their diagnoses moot and impossible if a home visit by the physician ever happened; in return, we have sacrificed the physician's personal "one on one" care.

Scientifically oriented medical healing tends to exclude anything dealing with subjective feelings, for the simple reason that moods or feelings cannot fit into a test tube. They are difficult to measure, categorize, label and evaluate, and then diagnose and treat.

Physicians responsible for correctly diagnosing patients' illnesses feel they need to go directly to the patients' health problems without having to deal with their emotional complexities. Medical doctors focus scientific technicalities of healing toward the patient and tightly adhere to what they learned in medical training; there is little mention of dealing with patients' emotions in medical school.

Discounting patients' emotions and neglecting to account for their opinions regarding their health conditions exemplifies the notion that physicians possess unshakeable "expertise" in which patients are passive recipients, unable to contribute towards their own healing. One patient explained that after all the tests, needles, trips to hospitals, and whispered conferences she felt like shouting, "BUT WHAT ABOUT ME! I'm still here in this body...what about me?" This is a common reaction with many patients who feel they have no say in their well-being, their mental well-being or their treatment as a human being. Traditional medicine tends to exclude subjective human emotions for the simple reason they consider moods or feelings "too messy."

Perhaps the most vital research on the subject of how emotions can affect physical well-being was done by Dr. Herbert Selye, who is in private practice in Maryland. Dr. Selye claimed the body is capable and well equipped to maintain itself in health, to cure itself of disease, and to remain youthful by successfully coping with factors which bring on "old age." These factors oriented from individuals' attitude toward life, which includes their spiritual activity. It appears that churchgoers and those involved with the daily practice of prayer are more likely to be happier and healthier than those who are not involved with spiritual activities. Those who are willing to forgive others and dissolve grudges, are less critical and less demanding are healthier than those who are not. Not being able to shrug off hurts and grief laid on us by our loved ones sends us down the road to disaster; forgive and forget is truly soul medicine... it cures the heart, mind and body.

Religious leaders more often outlive those involved in the medical or political field. The late Catholic pope, in his eighties, maintained a schedule that included traveling the world. His energy and vitality surpassed men much younger than he. His missions of spreading peace to the world kept him going. Other groups of people known for their longevity are those in the arts, particularly music. Creativity comes from the soul; it nourishes it, and keeps it active. Orchestra conductors tend to live to ripe old ages, Leonard Bernstein being an exception; a stressful private lifestyle contributed to his demise. No doubt, the subject of stress having a detrimental effect on one's health is apparent in all occupations.

CHAPTER 25

MORAL ISSUES

A MEDICAL DISGRACE

Regional Medical Center Bayonet Point in Hudson, Florida, recently suspended nine doctors for conduct unbecoming a professional. It is rare that a doctor has been suspended and even more rare to hear the plural being suspended. The case brought against the doctors—"Performing Unnecessary Surgeries." In this situation, these cardiologists were performing angioplasty to treat clogged arteries. Upon further examination of the doctors involved, discovery indicated the clog in the patient's arteries was not large enough to constitute surgery. The hospital is currently seeking patients who suffered this unnecessary surgery for damage. The investigating committee questioned the cardiologists why they chose surgery above instructing their heart patients about diet and exercise in controlling or eliminating the clogged artery.

Angioplasty surgery is performed in Canada and Europe as a last resort, but in the U.S., it is the first suggested and performed in greater frequency. In a seven-year study at University of Connecticut, under the COURAGE program, evidence discovered that angioplasty resulted in unnecessary complications and the hospital death rate is about one percent; a small percentage of patients suffer heart attack during the procedure. A much more common problem is resetenosis, a blockage in the treated artery that can send up to forty percent of patients back to the hospital for a repeat procedure. Bypass patients have a twenty-four percent risk of dying in the hospital and a five percent chance of suffering another heart attack or stroke during surgery. There is also a considerable risk of memory impairment, especially with patients seventy years old or older.

Cardiologist Prediman K. Shah, MD, director of cardiology and of the Arteriosclerosis Research Center at Cedars-Sinai Medical Center in Los Angeles, suggests a comprehensive non-invasive approach that can reduce heart attack risk as much as eighty percent. His recommendation includes following a Mediterranean-style diet, which is low in saturated fat and rich in omega-3 fatty acids found in fish. Diet and exercise increases the heart's efficiency, lowers blood pressure, boosts protective HDL cholesterol and accelerates the formation of collateral blood vessels that reroute blood flow around narrowed arteries. Dr. Steven Nissen, cardiologist at the Cleveland Clinic cardiology department, calls diet and exercise the prevailing "fireman mentality," and says that it is seldom offered to heart surgery patients as an alternative to surgery.

Alternative healing focuses on preventive measures regarding heart conditions rather than resorting to surgery or drugs; it is recommended that applying natural healing, such as focusing on change of lifestyle, a strict diet and exercise, be considered; medical costs will be minimal compared to other procedures. These alternative health measures can deprive some health professionals of their financial status. Surgeries bring enormous amounts of money to the medical establishment; thus surgery becomes first choice of most surgeons, placing their standards and medical ethics on the back shelf where they can, with little or no conscience, exhibit their financial enrichments.

Many stories tell of doctors being accused of some kind of health negligence. Lawsuits of malpractice have risen by leaps and bounds. Many patients, either from not knowing their rights or from being intimated by the powers of the medical field, usually do not proceed with legal action against their physician; if they did, lawsuits would skyrocket.

TESTIMONIAL

Several years ago, the artist Mark Hannel was admitted in a hospital with a fifty percent chance of malignant polyp growth inside his left nostril. At the time, he was experimenting with spray paints in his artwork and preparing for an important exhibit in New York City. His suspicions that there was something wrong started when he began suffering headaches and sore throat, followed with a clogged-up nose. A polyp had grown inside Mark's left nostril. On questioning if the spray paint was causing the problem, his surgeon denied that being possible, adding there should be no reason to discontinue its use. Upon the advice of his doctor, Mark continued using the spray paint, but gradually his health grew worse.

Shortly after, Mark discovered an article on toxins in his art magazines, giving information that microscopic particles from airbrush painting were extremely toxic when inhaled. The article advised to wear the government-recommended OSHA mask that factory workers use when working with toxic materials. When Mark brought this information to the attention of his doctor, the doctor was unwilling to accept the information and said, "It lacks scientific proof." This doctor's excuse is common when they want to avoid complex questions or statements made by patients that they have no interest in pursuing, or they have little or no knowledge of the subject at hand. Doctors, most often, will go into great detail how illnesses just happen or they are inherited from a past ancestor and their only job is to fix the problem. If you feel that your doctor is not being up-front with you, do the research, it can potentially save your life and prevent future illness.

NON-CARING COMES IN MANY FORMS

Indifference and non-caring comes in many forms. A caring mother with many children gives love to each as if each were an only child, whereas a non-loving mother with just one child can give all her attention to this one but treats that child as though she has twelve children. A good example would be a caring teacher who, regardless of her class size, recognizes the individual needs of each student and enjoys her role in serving these young people. A teacher with less-endearing qualities, who perhaps considers her position as unrewarding, grudgingly faces her children each morning. When non-caring is evident from a health practitioner the damage is more severe. During illness, one is more vulnerable, more at the mercy of the healer...the healer is regarded as the savior, perhaps able to restore health, even life to the patient. Too often, patients are faced with harassed, overworked, bored or arrogant practitioners who express minimal concern regarding their feelings and sensitivities, resulting in damage to the patient.

Rarely do we see traditional physicians calling on their patients, or checking on their well-being. Since this does not bring money to the physician's pocket, they do not even bother to call and check on the patient's well-being and if they do, the patient is billed for the phone call. When Dr. Danial Mayer, a chelation therapist, was invited to call the well- known Dr. David Perlmutter, a physician in Naples, Florida, who runs the chelation clinic to discuss their practice of chelation, Dr. Mayer was sent a $95 bill from Dr. Perlmutter for the privilege of the phone conversation.

When a doctor's office does makes that so-called "care" phone call the patient is surprised, but accepts the call with good cheer and pays the bill without question. Everyone likes to feel that their health care provider cares enough to make that follow-up call to check on their health or to see if they are taking their prescribed medication as instructed and if there are any side effects that would require him or her to change, strengthen or lessen the medication. It is ironic that "personal care giving," more often than not, is practiced only by non- traditional healers.

Dr. David Minkoff's Lifeworks Wellness Center makes it a habit to follow up with his patients regarding their well-being, knowing the benefits their emotional well-being makes in their recovery.

Personal note: My recent encounter with a medical office's priority is just a sampling of what has become a growing problem in allopathic medicine. In a visit to a medical clinic, I was shuffled in and out of various departments, where indifferent lab technicians took my blood and made other checks on my physical body. One technician discussed her dinner menu with another technician, without even so much as a glance in my direction. Since such attitudes are so prevalent in medical practice, we have come to accept this kind of behavior as normal.

Discussing other patients' well-being in front of other patients should not be acceptable. In that same visit, a patient came into the clinic with profuse bleeding from a gash in his foot. Rather than rushing him in to see a doctor, certain insurance questions had to be resolved before the clinic would even accept him or allow him the privilege of seeing the physician. As this man's foot continued to bleed, paperwork was shuffled around between the staff while another attendant called the patient's insurance company to validate if the policy was current. I was shocked and troubled at this clinic's lack of concern for this patient's well-being and the direction their priorities pointed.

COMFORT FIRST

"Comfort always, cure rarely" was a motto of medicine in times long gone, when bedside manner was considered far more potent than any medicine. Now, in the movement that counters the impact of high-technology and high-turnover medicine, few physicians seek out this lost art of healing. They are spurred by a steady march of scientific findings that prove the linkage between emotions and physical illnesses. In a recent study conducted by the University of Minnesota on eighty-seven patients undergoing bone marrow transplants for leukemia, thirteen were found to be depressed, and twelve of those died within a year; in contrast, thirty-four patients who did not suffer depression were still alive after two years. Among patients who received strong family emotional support, fifty-four percent survived the transplant after two years, while among those denied family support, twenty percent did not fare as well.

In another study, 122 men were evaluated for the degree of optimism and pessimism they felt during the period of suffering a heart attack. Such a state of mind was determined to be a more efficient predictor of death from a heart attack eight years from the original attack than were any of the standard medical risk factors, including damage to the heart, artery blockage, cholesterol levels or blood pressure. Among the twenty-five most pessimistic men, twenty-one died after eight years, whereas out of the most optimistic, just six died. Dr. James Strain, a psychiatrist at Mount Sinai, studied "elderly patients" receiving mental care during their hospital stay for fractured hips, and discovered they left the hospital two days earlier than patients who did not receive the same care. Dr. Strain claims that "physicians should take into consideration their patient's emotional state when treating them for medical problems, even major health problems, which demand stringent clinical healing." Increasing medical studies prove without a doubt, a patient's emotional well-being can actually control the patient's rate of healing progression. Various scientists interviewed, cited as particularly convincing, a study conducted in 1990 at Stanford University, that women with advanced breast cancer, when in support groups, lived twice as long as those with equivalent illness and medication, such as chemotherapy, etc. Even in seemingly minor situations, such as hospital patients' feeling of well-being and lifted spirits, stemming from their visitors, friends and family, and receiving get- well cards and flowers, play a part in accelerating the rate of healing. Whereas, those denied these elements of mental healing experienced lowered spirits and depression, thus prolonging their hospital stay.

Another study conducted by a psychiatrist in determining how the emotions affect physical health was done by Dr. Gary L. Elders. He reported that individuals who suffer from chronic inhibitions and who keep problems bottled up result in a myriad of disorders other than emotional ones, including allergies, breaking bones, hives, stomach disorders, ulcers, chronic headaches, and colds. He reports that such afflictions work as an alarm system where the subconscious mind attempts to seek emotional release. Unable to find this relief through the individual's conscious mind, emotions become manifested in various illnesses through the subconscious mind, driving the individual into illness and accidents.

Children in the arms of their loving parents are apt to suffer less illness than those who do not receive parental comforts. Chronic illnesses often stem from unloving environments. Children raised in orphanages, who receive minimal attention, personal supervision, care and love, are more vulnerable to illness and experience more serious illnesses than those from loving homes, and if the home becomes stressful to the child, illnesses become more apparent and the child is sick more often and longer. Grandparents who live with the child or close by and who were at one time the peace givers and provided the lap for the child to hide and nestle into acted as therapy. Care giving by medical staff, parents or guardians helps to prevent and eliminate many illnesses stemming from stress, allergies, migraine headaches, loss of concentration, etc. Now with the separation of families, along with the loss of supportive grandparents, and security blankets, kids have to go it alone. Children are suffering more often from these emotional-physical afflictions than at any other time in our history.

WELL-BEING OF THE ELDERLY

Chronic depression is prevalent with older people; the basic cause being, the general attitudes our culture has toward the elderly. We are far from being a society that respects the wisdom of the aged; instead, aging is regarded as being almost a deadly disease. We are a society that spends billions of dollars on cosmetics, medications and surgeries that make us look and feel younger. Many dermatologists have oriented their business to various cosmetic treatments and plastic surgeries because the income is enormous and the demand for youthful appearance is even greater; treating various serious skin ailments has been put on the back burner.

Separation from families, resulting in losing a sense of purpose, adding to this feeling of sense of uselessness to the workings of society is an additional factor for elderly depression. In the past, the elderly played an essential role in the homestead, where survival required the participation of all family members. The elderly were often in charge of domestic duties and the children. Often due to their experiences, they were chosen as community leaders responsible for making important decisions. We need to ask why millions of elderly Americans have been sequestered from the workings of society. Do we not need this resource as much now as back in the days when their contributions were essential, particularly now that people live longer and are healthier in their aging years? Are we vulnerable to repeating past mistakes rather than taking guidance from those who already experienced life? Does our society function so well that we could not benefit from this additional resource? Do we remember the protests during the feminist movement, how women could add to our national resources by allowing them to contribute their skills to society? Seniors can be regarded as being in that category; they too should be part of such as movement, such as being regarded as beneficial resources to the workings of our society.

Family breakup, divorce, moving to a job location, unable or unwilling to take care of the elderly parents, are the basic reasons for the separation of the elderly from the family. Ironically, today with working moms spending little time with their children, grandparents' care would be so beneficial for both parents and children. Instead, millions of children are being raised by strangers in daycare centers or by babysitters. Some children welfare centers have tapped into various senior citizens resources for parenting children with no parents, or to working mothers who have little time or patience for their children. Older people can offer qualities often lacking in modern homes with working parents. Senior citizens can offer a variety of assistance to the young. They can instruct home and childcare skills to young inexperienced fathers and mothers. Retired businesspeople and executives can train in the skills of salesmanship, managing a business and executive duties. Being contributing members of society helps keep seniors actively healthy. Statistics record mortality and illnesses rates are lowered when the elderly are made to keep busy.

The stability and security from having a sense of roots in one's surroundings is nonexistent in modern society. Youth often feel disconnected from their families, community and from themselves. Americans, more than any other country, disassociate themselves from the past in their adoration for the new. The elderly could also act as a linkage from the past to the present, in their communication of certain past experiences to subsequent generations. Their expertise in various fields and with life in general could benefit many a novice and generate a feeling of continuity for our past heritage.

In conclusion, any form of human neglect repeats itself in various directions. More women are being violently attacked, hate crimes, as well as other crimes have risen, child abuse and neglect has escalated and violent abuse by women against men has increased tenfold. All are part of a disharmony chorus of humanistic deterioration regardless of race, creed, or age. The growing prejudices, almost to the point of antagonism, are very prevalent against older people. Too often, conclusions are made that they are too inept to be considered relevant to the goings-on in society. Social Security and Medicare has put their stamp of recognition out to society, telling us when one has reached old age and is no longer useful. A growing number of older women who are still in good health, who have outlived their husbands, are finding themselves having to work and they are able to do so. They have proven that attitudes towards the aged members of our society are pure mind over matter and should not be tolerated. Still, society, so prone to adoration of the young, has its stigmas and attitudes and will not change until forced to do so.

SENSITIVE TO CHOICE OF LIFE OR DEATH

The battle by individuals wishing self-choice for their own death has superimposed itself onto various laws pertaining to the subject; terminally ill patients, suffering from severe and constant pain, often feel guilty of the enormous hospital bills their family will be left to pay; this reason, among others, is responsible for some patients requesting their lifeline be turned off. Such wishes have faced obstacles with the legal system. One recent episode that tested this right to euthanasia was with a man undergoing minor surgery and when something went wrong with the anesthesia, left him brain dead and permanently unconscious. His wife had initially made a promise to him that she would never let him live in a vegetative state connected to artificial life support machines. Ironic in this case, this patient is a physician and understands the consequences of keeping a brain-dead person alive with machines and against their wishes. Being able to keep that promise to her husband took more than a year of court battles, costing her her job and leaving the thirty-six-year-old woman emotionally brutalized. She claimed it was a tumultuous psychological trauma having to plead for the death of the person she loved most in the entire world. When she requested that the life-support systems be shut off and her husband be allowed to die, the Westchester County Medical Center refused, forcing her to file the lawsuit. Shortly after the case ended, she was fired from her job as assistant professor of medicine at New York Medical College, which is affiliated with the hospital where her husband was being treated.

This woman's concerns for others with similar experiences led her to urge lawmakers to approve legislation to help inform people of their right to determine their own medical treatment through living wills and other advance directives that would legally enable spouses, children or legal guardians to speak for them if they cannot speak for themselves. A living will is not a guarantee that these instructions will be followed but it will give you legal ground if faced with a similar situation as the doctor's wife.

Putting a substantive living-will statue in place in Florida has been an ongoing challenge. Repeated efforts to amend the Life-prolonging Procedures Act so that living wills would be honored have resulted in protracted legislative battles that pit an individual's right to die with dignity against politicians, physicians and hospitals. Those whose premise is "while there is life there is hope" see the possibility of cure by a miracle, regardless of how remote it may be. Delaying death also delays the grief by family members. Then there is the internal battle, which includes the question of selfishness in keeping a loved one alive or ending it for the sake of the suffering victim.

The issue of morality and the caring of the sick cannot be overly emphasized. No doubt, experiencing any form of lack of well-being, either emotionally or physically, places one in a vulnerable position where others are depended upon to take care of certain needs. In essence, this loss of self-reliance weakens the spirit and minimizes self-determination to do whatever is needed to overcome afflictions.

Ideally, the position of the healer is not only to treat patients but also to instruct and motivate them to learn processes they can take to accelerate their healing. Unfortunately, too many physicians have turned healing into a moneymaking commodity, resulting in a scandal where various medical individuals were overcharging for services to Medicare, or listing costs of services not rendered. This greed is far removed from what we idealistically envision a medical system should be—that being, one that acts with benevolence and dedication to healing the sick.

We come down to the question of how a medical establishment, so imbedded with profit and power, can be transformed into a system that regards healing as a priority above financial gain. The closest we can come to such an ideal is the manner in which we approach our own health well-being. Taking a more active role in our healing by becoming more aware, we can become cognitive in every detail of the healing process we encounter in our lives, rather than act as passive bystanders. In a manner, this active awareness can help empower individuals to be more in command over their health and of those who treat them when they are in need. With this, all healing processes need to be executed in consideration of ethics and morality, and needs to be the predominant standards of those dealing with healing.

CHAPTER 26

LOOKING TOWARDS THE FUTURE

It is difficult for institutions imbedded with decades of stringent traditionalism to accept new ways of doing things. One factor causing resistance towards alternative growth, ironically, derives from the younger generation. This group with their rushed and hectic approach to life often leaves minimal incentive in exploring alternative ways of doing things. Taking time to patiently learn and experiment is often scrapped for instant gratification. While at first glance, we may associate the younger generation with acceptance of alternative concepts, however, preoccupation with daily survival and tendencies towards focusing on the quick and easy, which may just mean avoiding having to take the time required in making changes, perhaps in the seeking out the best, results in them lacking motivation to change.

The consequence of this void is that our future generations will lack the advantage of knowing about alternative healing and on basic healthy living because their parents are unable to teach it to them. Sadly, the widespread problem of obesity is the result of this negligence. Even with all the information available on this subject, it is alarming how many individuals are still unaware of it. Many of the young generation are still not knowledgeable about supplements and herbal cures; instead they are popping pharmaceutical drugs and remain reluctant to venture into any form of healing outside the confines of traditional medicine. It is interesting to note that women approach this subject more actively than men do and many alternative healing practitioners are women.

Since physicians know little or nothing about alternative healing and they politely refuse to devolve what they do know, you take a chance in getting the wrong information. There are many books written on this subject and the expanding availability of such practitioners makes it simpler to learn anything you want to know. Visit your local health food or herb store that sells herbal medical books, ask for the book that gives the most thorough information on the subject you want to learn and then learn how to maintain your good health and well-being yourself.

See how much you are willing to expand your thinking regarding alternative healing in the questions listed below.

1—How much do you know about Chinese herbs, acupuncture, massage therapy, spiritual healing, mind and body healing, etc.? Have you experienced any of these healing modalities?

2—What is your level of belief in each? Do you have a particular health or emotional problem you may consider using one of these alternative therapies to heal?

3—Have you gone as far as searching for a practitioner who may offer such therapies?

4—Are you willing to take the time to do research to discover nontraditional means of healing the mind, body and spirit?

5—Do you believe you will find it difficult to break away from past methods of healing to find new ways? Are you truly willing to take a strong role toward maintaining your well-being, mind, body and spirit?

6—If you are suffering from a particular problem, is the healing method you are using helping? How concerned are you about the possible cause of the illnesses you are or have experienced?

7—Do you have a sense that something is wrong but your doctors cannot determine what it is? Are you frustrated because doctors have conflicting diagnoses for your ailments?

8—Do you feel your health is not what it should be? If so, do you feel helpless in doing something about it?

9—Are you truly prepared to make changes in your health care? Do you understand the concept of alternative healing. If not, are you willing to learn?

Ultimately, alternative healing is more comprehensive because it delves into both internal and external well-being of patients, their emotions, lifestyles, individualistic sensitivities, and spiritual outlooks, as well as physical well-being. Such a holistic approach to healing may appear to be very subjective; however, no more so than how doctors are aware that instilling their patients' trust in them helps to determine the success of their treatment. A physician can give patients a placebo (sugar pill) and most often, the patient will get well.

This "placebo effect" is so potent that a research survey done by F. J. Evans in 1974 revealed that the ingestion of the placebo "medication" can significantly reduce pain and suffering in approximately one out of every three patients. However, the trick is that a patient needs to have unquestioning confidence in the person who administers the pill. No doubt, this tells us how the emotions can dictate human behavior regarding their physical well-being. Subjective healing (placebo healing) incidents that because pf the physician's status, and a sugar pill, patients can be healed. The more assertive the physician's assurance, the more patients believe, the more certain the cure. Part of this is that patients want to believe their doctors' ability to cure them. In such situations, patients' emotions are mostly responsible for their healing rather the physicians' technical skills.

WORKOUT

(Self-analysis that will help in your search for alternative health care)

1—You have not been successfully treated for a certain illness by any traditional healing methods and still suffer from a chronic illness.

Perhaps you are on several drugs that may have side effects, causing you even more health problems.

2—Your doctor insists you take a drug for curing every illness and never mentions changing your diet or other healthy lifestyles. If you have high cholesterol, you may have been prescribed one of the new drugs on the market and not told to try a more natural approach, such as supplements or an herbal medicine like policosanols, coenzyme Q10—(a powerful antioxidant), alpha lipoic acid, grape seed extract, etc. If you are a diabetic patient, an alternative healer would prescribe chromium picolinate; if suffering from fatigue, the natural healer would recommend a nutrient-rich green super food for cellular health and energy, such as spirulina.

3—Your doctor does not discuss means to avoid future ailments, such as avoiding certain foods in your diet, or initiate a regime of exercise, or offering suggestions on methods to slow down your stress level, and also refrains from discussing possible reasons why you became sick in the first place. If you are prone to getting chronic sinus infection, you could focus on building up your immune system and learn how to minimize factors that lower the immune system.

4—You have been able to tap into the many facets of alternative healing which are now available. This resource has been growing by leaps and bounds, in which there are many alternative healers available in the field. To start, you can go to a good bookstore and read about holistic health and alternative healing. The most current information is provided by authors such as Gary Null, PhD, Andrew Weil, MD, and Elmer M. Cranton, MD; read Cranton's book called *Spontaneous Healing*. The next step is making that commitment to seek out alternative healing. There is plenty of information available that just didn't exist a couple a decade ago. New natural healing remedies keep developing and are readily available in most areas. Nothing is more important than taking time to make as many discoveries as you can in the field of natural healing and make a commitment in using them.

The following is a list that summarizes the essence of alternative healing:

1—Humans are dynamic energy systems which reflect evolutionary patterns of soul growth. The human consciousness is forever evolving in learning and growing. As this dynamic concept becomes recognized, it will change the essence of the nature of healing. Our health institutions will become places of wellness rather than places of illness. The medical establishment will focus more on how individuals can remain healthy rather than focusing on how to keep patients sick or overbilling their insurance company.

2—Patients will minimize their dependence on doctors to heal them. They will take their health into their own hands and take more responsibility in learning preventive measures of remaining well.

3—Illnesses are often a manifestation of individuals' sense of internal emotional conflict and spiritual blockage. As we age, we become more susceptible to emotional deterrents breaking down our immune systems.

4—Disease can be a sign that some kind of mental or physical constriction exists somewhere in the body or mind. The natural flow of the creative consciousness and subtle life energies through our multidimensional body/mind/spirit complexes may be negatively subjected to some external situation. Disease is a warning that something has become imbalanced; the constricted area needs cleared in order to restore health.

5—To clear these constricted areas, individuals need to consider practicing the chakra healing process listed in this manual. Going through this process should be consistently practiced regardless of whether you have a disease. Keeping the chakras cleared and well balanced will perpetuate good health.

6—Pertaining to chakra healing, none is more important than the lesson of the heart chakra. The opening of this chakra enables individuals to reach out and freely express themselves. It is the very soul and basis of the chakra system. If for some reason the heart chakra is blocked, energy and health diminishes. Releasing the heart chakra helps to rid the mind of fear and stress, two conditions which are the root of illnesses. When the individual acts from a higher plane, health and well- being evolve. Here we can see the direct relationship between emotions and physical health.

REVIEWING

An illness can act as an alarm system, offering information when an imbalance exists somewhere within the individual's lifestyle, be it physical, emotional or spiritual.

With this kind of self-awareness, one can be more responsible for his or her role in what to pursue in maintaining health. Alternative healing focuses on the process of determining cause and effect. Since each illness is a result of a particular distinctive cause, the key is to recognize the link between the two. When individuals are in tune with their bodies, such connections are obvious.

Listed below are some criteria for determining what alternative doctor or practitioner is right for you:

1—Doctor and staff express patience, concern, and treat you as an individual rather than just as another patient. Make sure you get a full comprehensive consultation and that you thoroughly understand the treatment you are inquiring about. Much information is available on the Internet, such as dissertations, explanations, testimonials from those who underwent treatments, and even information on those who did not benefit from such treatments. Make sure your holistic healer understands your medical concerns. You know your body, its strengths and weaknesses, so do not hesitate to add your knowledge and concerns of any given situations.

2—Beware of practitioners who promise too much; be careful not to be too vulnerable and too quick to accept promises of overnight super cures, or that the holistic healer is able to do everything and anything. Even in the alternative healing field, there are dishonest so-called "healers." Stick with known healers, get referrals, and make inquiries before making a decision.

3—The practitioner is willing and able to answer your questions over the phone rather than have you transmit them through the staff. If the doctor is too busy to answer your questions, he or she is too busy to have you as a patient. Some doctors in alternative medicine do have e-mail where patients can write in their questions.

4—Make sure this practitioner is practicing a healthy lifestyle himself. It is a good idea to observe the health condition he or she is in and they practice what they preach. Nothing is worse than an overweight practitioner who smells of tobacco or has heavy bags under their eyes due to a questionable lifestyle. Your healer needs to adhere to a good healthy lifestyle so he or she is believable when you confront them with your health concerns.

5—A practitioner or doctor who is willing and able to discuss integrating natural healing methods and change of lifestyle with you rather than automatically write out a prescription is worth your attention. Make sure this healer is not too set in his or her ways and is willing to keep up with the most recent alternative healing data. While most doctors treat ailments after they occur, some are learning to focus on prevention measures and are instructing these measures to their patients.

6—Do your research and find out what alternative healing methods have unfolded to the public in the last several years…acupuncture, massage therapy, chelation, spiritual healing, hands-on healing, Reiki, yoga, Chinese herbal medicine, NAET allergy testing, in Shin Do and many others.

The numerous treatments for just "pain control" include acupuncture, acupressure, biofeedback, chiropractic, guided imagery, heat and cold therapy, herbs, hypnotherapy, massage, meditation, relaxation techniques, and TENS unit therapy. With all these variable remedies, many that are fairly new in the healing field, it is a good idea to scout the Internet to research individuals in various healing fields located near you. You may find that some experts in the field may live a distance from you. If you are truly concerned about getting the best-quality treatments, you may have to do some traveling, particularly if you live in a rural area or district that lacks such innovative wellness treatments.

7—Take the time and correctly determine what therapy will benefit your current problem the most. It is best to find a good general health person, one that practices natural healing, before you decide on a specialist that specializes in areas such as acupuncture, homeopathic treatments, treating immune and toxic conditions, etc. You may even be able to find a medical doctor who is practicing in this field. Get advice from the practitioner as to what special treatments you should be getting for your particular health problem. As in the traditional medical field, holistic healing has its specialists. You may acquire a list of such health individuals in your area from the Internet. Make sure you thoroughly check them out, getting their references, testimonial information from prior patients, individual medical and certification boards, licenses, and just word of mouth. You do not want to spend big bucks on "fixes" that do not work.

8—Make certain the place you choose for your healing is well organized. You want your records kept in order and available to you if you need them. You want a means of following your progress of treatment and rest assured that you are being correctly charged for treatments. Obviously, some alternative treatments are expensive and not covered by insurance. Check to see what is covered by insurance through your medical physician, such as blood tests, then take these insurance-paid tests to your alternative healer. I have my family medical doctor give me my blood tests, paid by my insurance, and then if she writes a prescription for an ailment, I quickly run to my alternative healing clinic and get treated with supplements and other natural healing methods, depending upon my ailment. I have not had a cold in fifteen years and I am around children all the time. When I feel I'm getting the sniffles,

I quickly go on my regime and kick the bug out. In the meantime, I am taking immune-building substances to prevent future bugs.

9—Always try to keep up with treatments if you find them beneficial.

If you feel they are not working, talk it over with your healer and do not hesitate in seeking other health means.

10—Keep your knowledge up-to-date on the kinds of treatment you are seeking or currently getting. Many books on various healing methods are available, written by experts in the field, and the Internet is loaded with information. The more you know, the more you are in control over your process of healing and the better you can make your choices. If you feel it would be beneficial, you can add information that you have read or heard about; do not hesitate in discussing it with your healer. There will be times when health practitioners will disagree with you and even with each other. Since so much of alternative healing is new, even in its experimental stage, and much of it has not gone through the rigors of years of use, often definitive conclusions on healing methods are still questionable. The more you can learn and stay on top of the more you control will have over your healing process.

Alternative practitioners certainly do not know everything and they are still opening up the books and learning new material. You will find that these groups of healers are more involved with current research than traditional doctors, who often feel they have already gone through the rigors of training and there is nothing new for them to learn. Alternative healers tend to be more open to learning new healing methods.

Those seeking alternative healing are often desperate and search for any means they feel will magically heal them. This leaves them vulnerable to possible dishonest or inexperienced health individuals. I cannot stress this enough…always do your research and approach your healer with your head full of knowledge.

Choosing a medical doctor that practices alternative healing is the ideal situation (if you can find one) since you can rest assured he or she has a professional medical background. This is not saying a medical doctor is better in the alternative field; they could be better at diagnosing your problem. Medical doctors are easier to check on than are alternative practitioners since doctors are members of the medical board and there is more information at your disposal. Then from there you can check up on the various associations in the fields they practice. If the doctor practices acupuncture, allergy elimination, chelation, etc., check with these associations. A list of alternative healing resources can be found in *Nutritional Healing* by James F. Balch, MD, and Phyllis A. Balch, C.N.C. Many books on natural healing include the names of various healing associations. Look for health lectures at your library and bookstores, search by authors who have written on the subject; health food stores and various health clinics are also a good place to research your ailment or check on your health care provider. Lectures provide much firsthand information about health practitioners in various specialties. Lectures are also a good way to be introduced to a particular healer and their method; doing your homework will offer beneficial results. Ask questions and demand answers; after all, you are dealing with the most vital aspect of your life...your health.

Although physicians play an important role in modern medicine, total dependency on them for one's physical well-being minimizes the responsibility over your health. Such dependency denies one the ability to detect and to be in control over the various sensitivities, the subtleties so often overlooked that link causes and effects of one's state of health. The use of such healing tools as listening to one's own body, to one's senses, to one's inner voice and also listening to one's own heart, feelings, beliefs, instincts, and intuitions can act as vital resources in giving off messages that can reveal the direct source of what is causing a particular illness.

That is why health care needs to reconsider its present-day attitude towards ailing patients. Medical practitioners need to consider that patients are sensitive human beings, and fare better when treated holistically. Trained medical people may have difficulty understanding the holistic approach since "old-ways medical school" does not teach it. Changing times are so evident in the technological world that advances have grown by leaps and bounds. New healing concepts are expanding and emerging from the nontraditional healing field. Many discoveries indicate cures for diseases do not always have to come from a test tube; there are other resources available. To implement the ideals of twenty- first-century medical science into our society, all facets of healing, from medical science to alternative healing, need to be explored. All healing fields need to account for human beings' many layers of intricate complexities, some of which are still unfamiliar to the medical professionals, and they need to recognize that the human psyche directly affects individuals' physical well-being. This means that different healing methods need investigated and integrated into the medical field to improve the healing process.

Healing methods focusing on patients as human beings over medical science will enable patients to receive healing treatments that are more comprehensive and more holistic. This means integrating for emotional and spiritual concerns of the patient. Healers who use a more humanistic approach understand the importance of expanding their concepts and beliefs in healing; out of this blossoming, more seeds can be sowed in the field of *Preventive Healing*. Rather than attempting to heal individuals after the breakdown of their bodies and health, doctors will focus their attention to strengthening the immune system, thus keeping it vital so it can ward off the illness before it gets a strong hold on you. This will be a complete turnaround from present-day healing attitudes where the doctors treat patients only after they become sick and rarely prescribe preventive healing.

Part of the changes envisioned to manifest healing in the twenty-first century include doctors seeing themselves as healing gurus; guiding patients to live healthier lifestyles and maintaining good health to prevent illnesses. Emphasis will be on returning to various ancient healing methods, or to primitive natural healing, that regards healers as shamans, utilizing herbal cures, and spiritual healing methods. The ideal situation would be integrating ancient healing methods with modern medical technology to establish a well-balanced healing system where diversity in healing practices is available to every patient…trust and conviction by all parties need to be established and maintaining a deep moral sense and compassion from those taking on the responsibility of healing. Financial profiteering by the medical establishment and the pharmaceutical companies is immoral and criminal and must be eliminated. Included is the fact that the medicines and the many inefficiencies of the present-day medical profession make it too dangerous to continue on its own. Implementing alternative healing methods into the current medical field will bring more stability and more benefits to the healing industry.

Ultimately, the best solution for individuals who want to integrate alternative healing with the orthodox medical field is by exposing your allopathic physician to more homeopathic suggestions, which offers a multitude of healing benefits. Until medical institutions become less self- serving and take on a more active role serving humanity, medicine will be the most altruistic and heroic act humans will face in our modern-day society. Until medical professionals start conducting themselves in an honorable and noble way, healing will not reach its ultimate height.

Prisms of light are peeking through where rays of hope are shining new light in healing. Changes in healing for the twenty-first century should be a concern for everyone, including taking more responsibility for their own health and learning the many facets of alternative healing. Hope is that this manual will serve not only as a resource of information on the subject of alternative healing but also act as a motivating factor for initiating research in the field that will get and keep you healthy. Like any change, blockage in the road may exist and contain many obstacles; those dedicated to seeking out the most beneficial pathways to health and overcoming the obstacles that challenge us will benefit the most. Using this manual as a guide will ease the journey and ultimately offer end results responsible for helping to change present-day attitudes toward healing and help save lives without the use of doctors and medicine.